D1610512

C016148337

Nina Edwards is a writer and cultural critic, whose books include *On the Button: The Significance of an Ordinary Item* (I.B.Tauris, 2012), *The Secret Life of the Allotment* (Noumenon Kindle, 2013) and *Offal: A Global History* (Reaktion Books, 2013).

'Clothes have a language that illuminates the social and cultural significance of the circumstances in which they are worn. This is particularly true in wartime. *Dressed for War* is a fascinating and immensely readable account of in what and how both the military and civilians dressed, during the First World War. An apparently trivial subject turns out to have a profundity that adds a rich dimension to our understanding of the Great War in this its centenary year.'

Juliet Gardiner

DRESSED
FOR WAR

Uniform, Civilian Clothing
and Trappings, 1914 to 1918

NINA EDWARDS

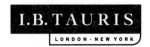

LONDON · NEW YORK

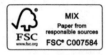

First published in 2015 by I.B.Tauris & Co Ltd
6 Salem Road, London W2 4BU
175 Fifth Avenue, New York NY 10010
www.ibtauris.com

Distributed in the United States and Canada Exclusively by Palgrave Macmillan
175 Fifth Avenue, New York NY 10010

ISBN: 978 1 78076 707 9
eISBN: 978 0 85773 511 9

A full CIP record for this book is available from the British Library
A full CIP record is available from the Library of Congress

Library of Congress Catalog Card Number: available

Printed and bound in Sweden by ScandBook AB.

To Sally Laird   1956–2010

CONTENTS

ILLUSTRATIONS

ACKNOWLEDGEMENTS

This book has relied on a wide range of scholarship and on the first-hand records of those who experienced the war. With thanks to the Bayerisches Armeemuseum Ingolstadt, Rod Hamilton of the British Library, the Museum of the Great War of the Pays de Meaux, the Historial de la Grande Guerre Museum Péronne, Helen Mavin and Katherine Phillips of the Imperial War Museum, Katherine Baird and Pat Cryer of the London College of Fashion, Simon Murphy of the London Transport Museum, Gerhard Bauer of the Militärhistorische Museum der Bundeswehr Dresden, the Museum of London, Emma Lefley and Nat Wieczorek of the National Army Museum London, the National Art Library at the V&A, Frank Arthur at the Royal Artillery Museum Woolwich and The Great War Forum. I would like to thank my editor, Philippa Brewster, whose idea this was and all at I.B.Tauris. Thanks to Sarah Aylen, Suzanne Barr, Angela Clark and Jenny Curtis of the British Button Society, Lizzie Bisley and Oriole Cullen of the V&A, Tanya Britton and Jonathon Oates of Ealing Libraries, Miodrag Certic, Josie Floyd, Vanda Foster of Gunnersbury Museum, Andre Gailani of *Punch* magazine, Ralph Gould, Philip Grimwood-Jones, Hove Museum, Tess Hines and Lucinda Moore of the Mary Evans Picture Library, Alastair McCartney of the Wellcome Trust, Lesley Manning and Colonel Frank Arthur Manning, Sheila Perkins, Patrick Quinn, Jane Reddish, Somerset County Library, Kate Swan, John Vassallo, Carole Walker. To Oliver Leaman for reading an early draft, and to Jeremy and Peter Edwards.

My very grateful thanks to the Society of Authors for a grant towards the completion of this book.

INTRODUCTION

Imagine a short silent film of the First World War. Seen from above, there are trenches and a desolate no-man's-land beyond. German cavalry in *ancien regime* spiked leather helmets are marching down the *Unter den Linden* boulevard in Berlin, and the women call out to them, reach out to them; in Trafalgar Square in London, a crowd of young men still in civvies throw their boaters in the air, like a flock of birds taking wing; a man in a backstreet bar in Paris, a little the worse for wear with drink, slouches in his red trousers, the blue jacket with its red piping slung on the back of his chair, an arm about the slender waist of a dark girl in a V-necked white blouse, the soft bouffant of her hair dissolving into the sunshine. All are smiling, as if a great adventure were about to begin.

Suddenly the screen grows dark but you can just make out movement. Then you realize there are individual men squatting down in khaki or grey – it is impossible to tell – passing the grog around for courage, reading a letter one more time, fixing bayonets, adjusting helmets. The camera follows each

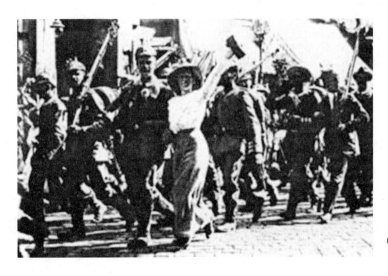

1. German recruits off to war.

1

one. From behind we cannot see their faces as they are ordered over the top. Like a magic trick, they are there and then they are not.

You see a field of poppies and now of graves, each marked with a small white cross. Old sepia photographs come to life, of grinning boys in uniform sharing a cigarette. A man in pilot's bonnet and leather coat leaning against a fragile biplane, his knee-length leather boots elegantly crossed at the ankle. A bluecoat sailor, in bare feet on gravel, runs with his rifle held out at arm's length. A group of Australian infantry, in wide-brimmed slouch hats turned up on one side, with their serge breeches cut short for the Gallipoli heat. They are quietly watching a boy, who looks 15, nonchalantly smoking a pipe with a long, curling stem, blowing circles for his mates to prove just how grown-up he is.

The film jumps to women in overalls belted over trousers, wearing rubber goggles, their hair in mobcaps, making shells or riveting together mechanical parts; women marching in khaki and navy blue, proud of their shapeless jackets and heavy boots; women in tented hospital wards with bloodied aprons, one nurse in a cardigan handing a handkerchief to a bandaged man on a stretcher. In Paris at the theatre, a girl in pleated, beaded silk fiddles with the bangle on her forearm, made from copper fuse wire from the Somme, for it is quite the thing. Her companion sits in a wheelchair in the aisle, a neatly folded blanket where the legs should

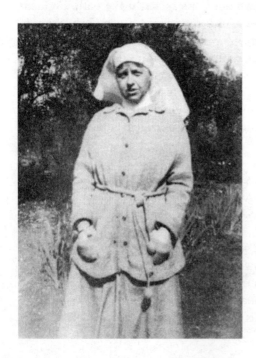

2. Edith Appleton nursing behind the lines.

be – a blanket manufactured from remnants of the uniforms of other men, too damaged to mend. Older women in long dark skirts, younger women with shingled hair and lipstick on, strain to read a list of names.

What people wear matters. This book examines what was worn for its significance, calling on what is revealed in the smallest details of personal dress, of clothes, hair and accessories, both in uniform and civilian wear, and in what comes in intimate contact with our bodies. During a period of extraordinary political, technological and philosophical upheaval, I want to suggest that a particular preference for a type of razor blade or perfume, say, the just-so adjustment to the tilt of a hat, the hidden fancy lining to a service jacket, and for the privileged, expensive trinkets such as, 'an officer's whistle in solid silver, which ingeniously combined a detachable compass and silver indelible pencil … [or] tinder cigarette lighters whose discreet glow was guaranteed not to attract the attention of the enemy if lit in the trenches',[1] – such diverse small things may begin to offer insights into the individual experience of that time. What such choices mean is seldom clear and the 'cues and clues'[2] can be half-hidden and open to different readings, but it is the intention here to uncover meanings that are peculiar to the study of dress.

Dress can be comforting or sometimes humiliating, it can divert or lead us headlong into new experience. Its dullness or uniformity can be distressing. A soldier, on frontline duty, his boots heavy with mud, his tunic spattered with a comrade's blood, was glad of a cheerful knitted scarf worn discreetly at the neck. A woman dressed in the armour of high fashion, took secret comfort in the unassuming narrow leather belt that had once belonged to a brother now missing in action. For some, clothing could be an affront to their principles. A sergeant, ordered to punish a conscientious objector by forcing him into uniform and leaving him in the open in freezing conditions till morning, is taken aback to discover that:

> During the night he [had] stripped himself of his khaki and shredded the whole of the suit up and hung it around the barbed wire, and that man [had] walked about all night long without a shred of clothing on him.[3]

The same sergeant is ashamed to forcibly shave off the beard of another conscientious objector. 'I shall never forget now his eyes as he looked at us, to think what we fellow men were doing to him.'[4] Clothes and an apparently small matter of personal grooming have become the means of one young soldier questioning his beliefs regarding a man's duty to fight for his country.

In contrast a soldier is made to wear outdated uniform as punishment, for asking to return home to his wife and pigs rather than go abroad to fight. He becomes an example of individual defiance:

> The colonel decided to shame [Probert], and he continued, by order, to wear the peacetime scarlet tunic and blue trousers with a red stripe … His mates called him 'Cock Robin'.[5]

The rest of his regiment is kitted out in temporary navy before their khaki uniforms arrive, while Probert remains in scarlet, spattered with grease from his kitchen duties. His mates call him Cock Robin, chanting a popular chorus of the time in his honour, 'In my old red vest I mean to cut a shine/Walking down the street they call me "Danger on the line!"'[6] Cock Robin has an echo of an older English nursery rhyme which asks who is to blame for a robin's death, and thus, by inference, who might be responsible for Probert's potential death in action.

What people wore had an effect on how they came to understand themselves. This was a period of rapid change, reflected in clothing, and to some extent new ways of dressing that in turn fostered change. When women began to wear what had previously been male-only clothing, and were criticized for giving up their femininity, this is reflected in the idea that such changes in gendered behaviour are evidence of modernity.[7]

Given the nature of any war, an oblique approach, examining its nature through the prism of dress, can be productive, for what we wear may be a peculiarly powerful signal and even at times an unwitting giveaway. Across Europe, at the outset of the war, crowds of civilians gathered to cheer on marching ranks of soldiers. They must have seemed brave and invincible. In the German town of Schneidemühl, not far from the Russian border, men were festooned with flowers, symbols of fragile, ephemeral beauty:

> All the soldiers had long garlands of summer flowers round the necks and on their chests. Bunches of asters, stocks and roses were even stuck into the barrels of their rifles as if they would shoot down the enemy with flowers.[8]

The 12-year-old girl who recalls this in her diary, Piete Kuhr, visits a hospital for wounded soldiers and is astonished to find that the men take comfort in such feminine things:

> Funny, isn't it? Men wanting flowers! … Later on I noticed that the badly wounded man was holding the flowers against his forehead; the leaves of the flowers helped to cool his fever.[9]

Flowers can represent political resistance. Following the German occupation of Belgium, the populace was forbidden to demonstrate, but:

> They had not forbidden the Belgians to wear flowers and the flower-vendors were out in force selling poesies of red and yellow blooms, which, worn in the lapel of a black frock-coat or pinned to a black dress, represented the colours of the Belgian flag. [10]

Conversely, black, white and red ribbon was made into bunting, coloured pompoms for buttonholes and to adorn children's hair, signifying German support for the war in August 1914. A milliner in Friedrichstrasse, Berlin cannot find enough ribbon to meet the demand. In Schneidemühl, Piete Kuhr is told by her teacher to wear ribbons on her shoes as well, but already she has begun to take stock of what war means. She watches the passage of soldiers to and from the Russian front, glimpsing the dishevelled prisoners of war and the wounded, as she helps her grandmother with Red Cross duties at their local railway station. Now she is less respectful, replying 'that I would even stick a bow on my behind'. [11]

An eager English recruit, expecting that war will be a noble experience, finds that uniforms are initially unavailable, so has to be satisfied with 'just a

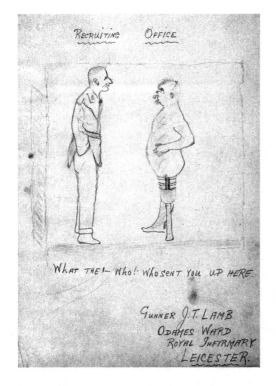

3. A satirical cartoon by Gunner J. T. Lamb of a recruiting officer with potential recruit.

square of card with the name of the Regiment stamped on, together with a bit of red, white and blue ribbon attached, and such was sufficient to proclaim to the world at large that we were members of the British Army'.[12]

It is not only the choices or adaptations made to dress, but also the textures, scents and resonance of clothing that can be as evocative as, say, the memory of a cake we once ate. The smell of damp, muddied wool, the crackle of starched linen, stained clothing soaking in a basin, sunlight catching the edge of a brass button or its impression as we happen upon it years later in a tin of odds and ends: such impressions can bring the past suddenly to life again. Sometimes an image or a memory, of hair and clothing, can evoke the past, as when a French soldier imprisoned in a Bavarian fortress longs for his wife:

> She is dressed in green. The dark perfume of her golden hair enwraps me.[13]

Sometimes civilian garb could seem a welcome distraction. A German soldier finds an item of clothing in an enemy dugout, and feels driven to put it on without delay:

> I strolled along the ravished trench ... The sight of a beautiful striped shirt, lying next to a ripped-open officer's valise, seduced me to strip off my uniform and get into some fresh linen. I relished the pleasant tickle of clean cloth against my skin.[14]

The experience has him for a moment consider the man to whom it had so recently belonged. Clothes can evoke the past by drawing you into the moment-to-moment experience of another: of a Salvation Army officer serving doughnuts in a bivouac, her coat a little too tight across the shoulder blades as she reaches forward; a Russian recruit, her hair shaved so close there is a rash at the nape of her neck; a pair of discarded German service boots with shattered cardboard soles. These visceral impressions help us imagine ourselves there with them, as them, in their shoes as it were.

Sometimes discarded clothing was worn simply because it was found to fit the bill, so that, for example, during the spring offensives on the Western Front, the 7th Bavarian Regiment commonly adopted British issue leather jerkins they came across in the trenches.[15] One German officer decries the looting that goes on at Rethel in the Ardennes, but admits:

> I couldn't resist taking a little memento myself here and there ... I found a splendid Aquascutum [raincoat] under [a] staircase and a camera for Felix.[16]

When I have been allowed direct access to stored 1914–18 uniforms,[17] and the great reverend boxes are laid out and the tissue pealed away, I touch the fabric through white cotton museum gloves, clumsy as a clown, and feel a sort of craving for that past time when these clothes were worn, sweated into, torn, bloodied, de-loused, scrubbed clean and mended to be worn again.

War is deeply connected to the material substance of living; to the conquest not just over land but over flesh and blood humanity. To understand how people experienced clothing then turns in part upon our view of the body, then and now, regarding sexuality and attitudes to contraception for example, to dentistry, to a sense of modesty and of display, a sometime desire for glamour, and lays bare the adaptations that had to be made in the light of horrific injury. The textural and associative oppositions of dress[18] provide interest and perspective for the individual and for society. For instance, standard British Army issue, machine-made socks were harder wearing and often more comfortable, yet a poorly knitted pair from home was often valued more highly for their nostalgic associations, for the sense that someone was thinking of them. Messages were often included with such gifts so that it was as if the anonymous donors became substitute sisters, mothers, sweethearts, who cared about them personally. Pat Barker[19] investigates the notion that officers took on a maternal role for their men, and in this context the doling out of small comforts, socks, scarves, cigarettes and various keepsakes, shored up a sense of familial intimacy.

Items of flamboyant dress that reassured the wearer of the past courage and style of his regiment, say, could seem more important than questions of camouflage in the psychological trauma of the firing line. The study of dress at such a time is not merely an investigative measure, but calls on the intrinsic value and sensual delight in what we wear, even in the theatre of war. Whether something feels alluring or dowdy can encourage or discourage. An item of clothing has the power to furnish distinct memories and to become part of what a person is.

***

On the home front, for both sides in the war, clothes had to be practical for new roles, to avoid, for example, a skirt catching in machinery or a corset so restrictive that a woman could not properly manage the labour required of her. In some cases, what had not been mainstream fashion pre-war was adapted to become more ordinary wear, as with the vogue for pantaloon trousers, which were modified to become both pyjama and more tailored trousers.

New roles had need of new dress codes. Even when it was just a matter of a new warm coat or serviceable footwear, choices again had to be made. For women, how to wear your hair and whether or not to be seen to wear make-up; for men, whether to grow a moustache or remove a beard, attitudes to appropriate garb in terms of class and age, of masculinity and femininity – all are revealed through the mirror of dress.

To explore these shifts and turnabouts, *Dressed for War* looks at changes in dress through its detail and nuance, and calls upon individual responses at the time. The war brought many women up sharp against their own deeply embedded notions of gender. Men too, in decrying the sight of a woman untidily or 'inappropriately' dressed say, had in effect to address a sense of their own masculinity, for it might have seemed troubling to witness women not primarily concerned with how they were seen.

At a time when the new middle classes, product of the Industrial Revolution, had already begun to threaten old class certainties, war meant that in some spheres the way people dressed was becoming harder to read. In Germany industrialization was more recent than in Britain, and a new optimism fuelled a hunger for consumer goods, including a desire for sumptuous new apparel among the up-and-coming classes. Theatre and music hall stars were the style icons of their day, at the cutting edge of fashion. Just as a gentleman might now look very much like a clerk, in his understated dark clothing right across developed Europe, the wartime working woman was dressed for practicality and a sense of cohesion. In jobs that involved hard labour such as factory work, women of all classes began to look very much like those working-class women who had always had to work for their living, sartorial distinctions sublimated to a common purpose.

There are, of course, many exceptions to this tendency, often revealed in small customizations, and one might argue that a refusal to conform absolutely to a common mode of dress betrays the survival instinct not only of class distinction at times, but also of fashion, which by its nature thrives on deviance.

Uniform, and the ways in which its permutations and eccentricities drew from and influenced clothing, have come to reinforce the uniform-like motifs in much subsequent design, from Yves Saint Laurent to Lady Gaga. The trench coat, Norfolk jacket for both genders, the American zipped flying jacket with its snug cuffs and waistband, stout laced boots and the knitted fatigue cloche are just some of the styles that have since become classics – forebears of today's beanies, hoodies, Doc Martens, forces' surplus-store gear and the gangster/Guantanamo Bay look.

Khaki and gabardine, leather and fur were given a new prominence. These materials were important, as we shall see, in providing adequate protection on the field of battle, but the ways in which they were taken up into civilian clothing show fashion not as amoral vanguard, but as aping, sometimes with sensitivity, what is most significant in the culture of the time.

Just as the high-fashion lady's bonnet of Victorian England (a tall, cylindrical cap, ornamented with gold braid, jewelled military-like badges and fanciful 'Vesuvius in eruption' plumes or wild silk pompoms) and the tasselled toque of the Parisian salons (in sugar-almond glacé leather or polished satin covered in stumpwork embroidery) echo the headgear of soldiers of the Crimea, the fashion for khaki in London and of field grey in Berlin did not denote disrespect. Rather the contrary. The influence of colonial troops' gear, for example, can be found in high fashion turbans, and versions of the Prussian shako returned to Berlin fashion even as it was in the process of being phased out as combat wear in the conflict.

Just as children's games became engaged with the war, fashion too plays out its influence. Versions of the uniforms of the First World War, in adult fashion and children's replica outfits, could not help but reference both gallant elegance, and also mutilation and death. The apparent playfulness is a way of confronting what is both serious and difficult. Clothing links these very different contexts, of giddy fashion and deadly combat, and in turn questions our connection to the material world, of bits and bobs, of apparently trivial ephemera. While dress might also be said to have offered, on occasion, a release from the single-minded necessities of warfare, even for those on the frontline, as you pull on a simple knitted hat you can be brought up sharp against its history, of a freezing soldier eating his rations from a mess tray or crouching low, under fire in a bivouac. Men might hope to look on war as an adventure, as an opportunity to cut a dash, but their experience of fear and boredom, horror and self-reappraisal, resilience and despair, is borne out through what was worn.

Despite the pressures on men of fighting age to be wearing uniform, there are accounts of the release they could feel on leave in civilian clothes again, reminiscent of children casting off their uniform at the end of a school day along with all their cares. The particular choices made of plus four golfing costumes or brocade dressing gowns ordered by post to await their return, of gifts bought from Parisian boutiques to send home to the Home Counties or the Steppes, of Belgian silk embroidered postcards in German or French, English or Russian, or of lace bought in Brussels for the Rhineland – such purchases represent an imagined future beyond the single-minded parameters of warfare.

Dress, from uniform to everyday civilian accommodations, to high fashion, has meaning for our interpretation of the First World War. In order to understand how significant those four years were, I want first to consider the prelude – the period that came before. In the first decade of the century the details of what people wore were still largely drawn along class lines, but the question is to what extent evidence of change made possible by industrialization was already apparent before the war had begun.

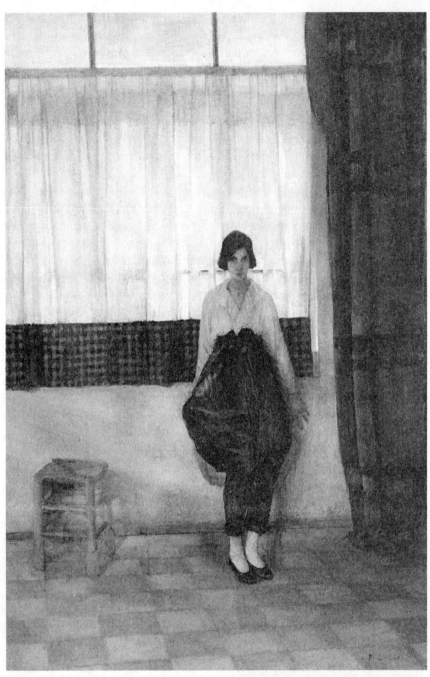

4. Self-portrait of the artist Madeline Green,
exhibited at the Royal Academy Summer Exhibition
in 1918, but painted at the war's outset.

1 THE PRELUDE

As the state of war gathered momentum across Europe, the step dancer leans back against a curtained window, the light of a new age like a halo surrounding her. The painting was shown at the Royal Academy Summer Exhibition in 1918, yet it is an image of optimism at the war's outset,[1] with striped green silk taffeta iridescent harem trousers, recalling Amelia Jenks Bloomer's enthusiasm for the eponymous loose trousers gathered at the ankle and worn under a short skirt, which had become briefly fashionable for ladies' bicycling in the 1850s. The woman in the painting wears a white blouse rather low-necked and feminine, in soft Pierrot-like folds. The hair is shingled, and on her feet are ballet slippers and white stockings, in homage to the costumes of the Ballets Russes, so recently arrived in London from Paris. This is the self-portrait of Madeline Green, a young middle-class English artist from a comfortable London suburb, and she looks out at us conscious of the effect her version of the exotic demands. It is daring, but not too daring. The mood suggests something of the *Perfect Summer* Juliet Nicolson evokes,[2] of indolent pleasure heightened by a vague sense of excitement ahead, of the aristocracy in tennis whites or toying with a croquet ball, too lazy to play in the late summer heat, bored but expectant.

Punch magazine, with its humorous often satirical approach, lampooned *The Step Dancer* from its high-status, male viewpoint, in a cartoon where the gentle gaze has turned shrewish, her stockings bagged around bony ankles and ungainly flat feet – with a deeper décolleté revealing a scrawny, hollow chest.[3] The message seems to be that pre-war modern girls are sexually uninviting and not remotely challenging.

A generation before and fashionable young women were tightly laced into steel framed corsets. The S-bend corset created a smoothly proffered mono-bosom and a tiny waist, that so-called symbol of beauty and femininity, exaggerating further the arching, bustled behind. Then, in a kind of deliberate opposition, she was buttoned primly to the neck, at least for daywear. Like Edna Pontellier in *The Awakening*, women's clothes are both forbiddingly up-holstered and yet give the impression of vulnerability 'with a fluffiness of ruffles

… [and] draperies and fluttering things'.[4] In John Singer Sargent's paintings, women with their opulent Gibson Girl curves, their rich brocades and velvets, seem larger than life. Hats were borne vast and festooned with flowers, swathes of curling feathers and veils of tulle, to balance out the hourglass figures beneath. In the evening women's chest and arms were suddenly laid bare, albeit unapproachable as marble statuary, in flimsy chiffon fabrics over the whalebone and steel corsets beneath, 'in obedience to the decorative instinct which calls for fine clothes in fine surroundings … a surface of rich tissues and jewelled shoulders'.[5]

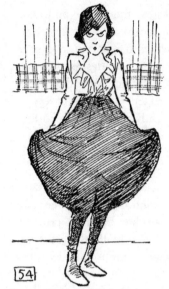

"I DON'T THINK I FEEL FUNNY ENOUGH FOR A CLOWN."

5. *Punch's* view of *The Step Dancer*.

This contrast is in some counterpoint to uniform, which seeks to make bodies appear invincible, even though beneath the carapace of hardwearing fabric, the leather and tough webbing belts and carriers, the stout boots and metal helmets, the tender flesh remains.

The transformational aspect of uniform might not always succeed in persuading the onlooker as to the wearer's character. An astute Piete Kuhr at 14 years old, courted by a dashing lieutenant in German Flying Corps splendour, considers his shoulder-pads and thinks that 'without his finely tailored uniform he might not look so handsome'. Some months later, however, she is disappointed by the lacklustre sight of her brother in the new less tailored field dress, 'Was this Gil? … in loose-fitting uniform with concertina trousers, thick boots and crazy-looking helmet? And his lovely soft, dark hair cut short? Oh Gil, my brother Willi!'[6]

The turn of the twentieth century was an age of richly detailed adornment for women – for those who could afford it – everything trimmed with lace, ruffles, velvet and fringe. Women's clothing might be elaborately embroidered in deference to the Aesthetic Movement, which was anti-modern in its outlook, its influence extending across Europe and the United States (which from now on will be referred to as America). Materials for those of means were extravagant and often impractical, with fine wool cashmeres and even shantung silk for day, figured cotton and silk muslins in summer and gossamer tissue and chiffon for evening. Longer-lined, boned bodices with more fitted skirts eschewed the need for layered petticoats, a glimpse of which had for so long suggested a hidden female vulnerability beneath. However, the design of women's clothes continued to constrict and many of the fabrics were deliberately high maintenance. Washable fabrics were associated with those of low status, who worked for a living.

Pre-Raphaelite Greco-Roman draped styles of the Arts and Crafts Movement appeared to give women more room to breathe, though it is significant that in many cases corsets continued to be worn unseen, Alexandra Palmer describing Jane Morris, for example, as having 'no lacing or corset *visible*.[7] It suggests that for many it was the appearance of having discarded traditional underwear that mattered, rather than the expression of genuine change, returning to some romantic notion of medieval simplicity. With their flowing lines and less demanding underpinnings, women's sumptuous dress still expressed either conspicuous wealth and/

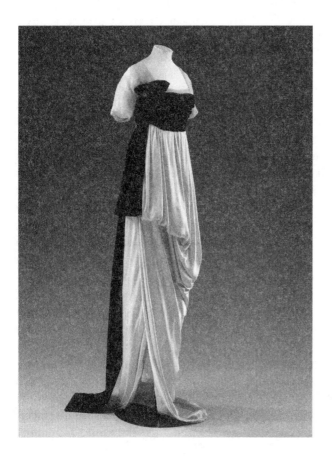

6. Satin evening dress by Lucile, *c.*1912, trimmed with chiffon and machine-made lace, silk velvet, lined with grosgrain and whalebone. This was described by the designer as 'so lovely that [it] might have been worn by some princess in a fairytale', *Discretions and Indiscretions,* 1932.

or created an illusion of an imagined past romantic age. Stella Newton describes the hand embroidery, so valued on artistic clothing, as not only inexpensive to produce at home, but significantly here that 'it could be *seen* to be of very little cost' (my italics).[8] The Arts and Crafts woman might ape medieval homespun accomplishment, but in reality her clothing was still made by a dressmaker in the main, a little light embellishment the extent of her involvement. When women did take on the making of their garments, then it tended to be as a hobby, supported by the wealth of a supporting male breadwinner.

A. S. Byatt depicts a Fabian circle in the late 1890s[9] playing at homemade costume as artistic expression, but underpinned by the confidence bred of class and economic security. One household takes the style too far. Seraphita Fludd has become eccentric rather than artistic with her fanciful dressmaking, betraying the moral deviation within her close family, coupled with its financial decay. C. Willett Cunnington reads a general moral decay into the turns of fashion at the dawning of the new century:

> Were the Suffragette Movement and its contemporary, the Hobble skirt, antagonists or queer products of a common impulse? In the darkening twilight of Class Distinction shadowy new forms were picturing the shape of things to come, the fashions and the events so mingled that we can hardly comprehend the one without the other.[10]

A connection is being made here between what appears to liberate women's clothing, and fashions that deliberately impede natural movement. Rational or reformed dress codes at the 1907 International Women's Socialist Conference in Stuttgart, for instance, were wide ranging, from Liberty-style loose robes to much plainer dress among some German and Dutch participants, and the British novelist E. Nesbit.[11] The fashion for these so-called new forms of dress was short-lived, Valerie Steele putting its failure to catch on down to women's fear of looking fat.[12] Cunnington describes a persistent anxiety as representing 'a pathetic reluctance to abandon all the devices of sex-attraction'.[13] He has little time for the 'sensible' clothing worn by many suffragettes, although the mainly well-to-do women drawn into the movement's ranks were often in fact fashionably got up, some pictured in what appears to be hobble skirts and huge, impractical and elaborately confectioned hats. When Emily Wilding Davison went under the king's horse at the 1913 Derby, she was kitted out in a soigné black tailored suit with a brooch in the purple, green and white colours of the movement, to match her splendid protest banner. Earlier photographs show her in *de rigueur* feather boa and broad-brimmed hat.

The relative colourfulness and variety in female clothing, as opposed to male solemnity, was a distinction that applied more to the upper and emergent middle classes, with the means to afford the impractical. For the working classes, for servants, shop, factory and office workers and for those who worked in the field – in America and particularly in less-industrialized Europe – for all those who laboured at cottage industries while caring for their offspring in the home, fashion was largely unaffordable and clothing was more often than not mainly plain and dark enough to forgive dirt and wear. Even a cotton print was a considerable extravagance, to be carefully budgeted. A fortunate lady's maid might inherit her mistress's cast-offs, and used clothing was traded down, but otherwise colour, pattern and choice of fabric was limited.

It took war to grant women across the board an opportunity to more fully engage in new shopping and fashion opportunities. The percentage of women working was not significantly higher during the war, 32 per cent of French women employed at the beginning of the war as opposed to 40 per cent in 1918, 26 per cent mounting to 36 per cent in Britain, and because of the sharp rise in women's employment in the two decades preceding the war, an actual decline in Germany.[14] Nonetheless it was the change in the nature of women's work and the resultant rise in women's wages that gave them more spending power. Women gained greater economic clout and thus a measure of autonomy to access fashion. Moreover, there was less stigma attached to women of all classes aspiring to fashion. Working collaboratively as never before, thrown together in armaments factories for example, in relation to both women's attitudes at home and those working near the frontline, women's dress across class boundaries began to look more alike.

As for men, the elaborate male dress of the eighteenth-century male, the velvet and silk coats, the lace furbelows and embroidered waistcoats, gorgeously painted and jewelled *passementerie* buttons, sparkling buckles and exquisite pale silk stockings, had given way to the nineteenth-century dandy, all refined monochrome in figure-hugging trews, carefully tied cravat and elegant tailoring. Now, in the first decade of the twentieth century, the Great Male Renunciation of display was fully entrenched. Men had retreated into their now familiar dark uniformity, so that it was difficult to distinguish class, status or even income from dress alone, plain dark clothing of superior quality making very much the same passing impression as the mass-produced.

Sarah Frantz, discussing Jane Austen's soberly dressed and reticent heroes, suggests that this denial of sumptuous dress demonstrates 'a similar renunciation[15] in men's ability to express their emotions'. She argues that 'men's dress, in order to symbolize power and self-control, was supposed to be unremarkable' recalling Beau Brummell's view that it was not seemly for a well-dressed man to turn heads. Any outward display might suggest weakness or effeminacy, and it is only lately that men have been able to express emotion in public without embarrassment, even on occasion appearing to raise their status as men thereby. At the outbreak of the First World War men were already largely dressed to avoid individual differentiation, as they sought to square up to the dangers ahead without either the show or even the experience of fear. To be proper men they needed to put aside self-interest: 'Steeled to suffer uncomplaining.'[16]

Uniforms are about the 'comfort and vanity of belonging';[17] war is a context where it is essential to work together to a common end. A Frenchman scorns German pride in uniform, 'Everywhere I saw blind adoration of the uniform, overwhelming joy in wearing it,' and dismisses German soldiers as 'a fine army of automata!'[18] However, as a prisoner of war (POW) he is evidently concerned to maintain his own uniformed appearance and takes delight in describing in his diary its many permutations amongst the French and Russian prison inmates.

The adoption of men's service uniform and its myriad adaptations, and the range of uniforms developed for women during the war, were important factors in the preparation of resilience under threat. Uniforms affected how people saw themselves and how they came to feel about their own inner life. They influenced the expectations of others. Women in uniform displayed, often by stealth and in small matters, a predilection for what was first and foremost aesthetically pleasing – but then so did men. The curious tension between the prescribed strictures of uniform, and its individual and group customizations echoes, as I hope to show, an ambivalence towards the state of war. Attitudes to clothing reveal what can be difficult to articulate by other means.

Women's Fashion

Prior to the First World War the fashion for the hobble skirt, with its revolutionary daring flash of ankle, meant that women's mobility was deliberately limited, with a tape fastened behind the knees, allowing for only the small tripping step of the geisha or bound Chinese foot. This deliberate assumption of physical disability was in some irony influenced by the costumes of Diaghilev's fluidly mobile dancers. Women were still doll-like, but exotic doll-like, and the skirts that hobbled their natural stride demonstrated their conspicuous leisure as deftly as today's killer heels. The lampshade tunic, with its loose kimono sleeves, after the Parisian designer Paul Poiret, became a staple layered silhouette, topped with a swathed turban perhaps, straight from the orient of Léon Bakst. Poiret was the first major couturier to use draped design over more traditional corsetry and

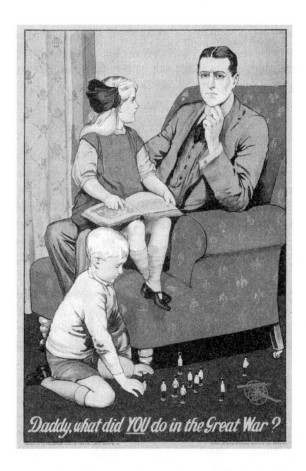

Daddy, what did YOU do in the Great War?

7. A British pre-conscription lithograph, 1914–15, by Savile Lumley. The father's civilian suit is set against the boy's uniformed toy soldiers.

tailoring techniques. When he signed up in 1914 the French army employed him as a tailor, drawing on his experience to simplify uniform production.

In the pages of *The National Fall and Winter Fashion Catalogue* of 1914, where clothes were orientated towards the middle-class market, there is a noticeable marriage between a softened version of the Edwardian hourglass silhouette and the exotic influence of Bohemian style. Its illustrations still display a low mono-bosom bust, but the waists have relaxed, with long tunics falling over a straight-ish underskirt. Hair is crimped, resembling a turban in shape. A simple *fichu* or bib, often of lace, makes modest the lower V-necks of the bodice. Such new low necklines were denounced by the clergy as immodest, and by the medical profession as risking pneumonia. The women wear buttoned boots, but usually with white gaiters. Hats have shrunk, sometimes with a small brim turned back with a feather standing straight up, or prim and flat as a Spanish priest's; several sport a sailor's cap in navy and white or more military looking wool cap, but all markedly different in impact to the arching peacock display of the Directoire show hat. It is as if women's headgear is in tune with the reservists marshalling on the city streets of Europe, women's clothing beginning to imitate Poiret's simplified army tunic designs.

***

Accompanying these mild translations of style, men are uniformly in dark square cut suit jackets and waistcoats, with often slightly contrasting trousers, pleated and worn with creases down front and back,[19] more often with turn-ups. For younger men, the more softly tailored lounge suit is worn with an accompanying Homburg hat, the central dent in its crown adjusted as it should be, though these were sometimes thought of as caddish by more conservative taste, and were more slowly adopted in Britain[20] than on the Continent and in America, where it suggested an urban nod to the cowboy Stetson.

The influence of sport was still evident, with simple blazers, bound with contrasting colour or brightly striped and matching a club or old school tie. Straw boaters for summer were popular across the board and small Tyrolean fancies, even hats decorated with 'huntsman' teddy bears after President Roosevelt, were fashionable. Tweed hunting jackets were worn for leisure time, with baggy plus fours and patterned knee socks.

For evening wear, men of society stuck to their dark tail coats and white tie with stiff, miserably constricting wing collars, in startling contrast to the flimsily dressed sultanas, Turkish slave girls or woodland nymphs their wives and consorts had become. By the end of the war, when many women had become accustomed to wearing uniform and uniform-like suits; their evening wear became in contrast even more markedly flighty, and it is this distinction, between day and evening, that led to evening wear becoming known as 'glad rags'.[21]

A subset are those few women able to take advantage of higher education in this pre-war period, dressing as if in deference to male style and thus status, in starched collars and college ties but with hair, still long and 'balancing like a satin cushion on each head'.[22] The bulk of women had little opportunity for education or for political pursuits such as the Suffragette Movement, but this was to change when men and women alike were thrown together in a common purpose.

Dress as a Catalyst

On 28 June 1914, on a visit to Sarajevo, Archduke Franz Ferdinand is filmed approaching the imperial motorcar with Duchess Sophie. He is wearing full

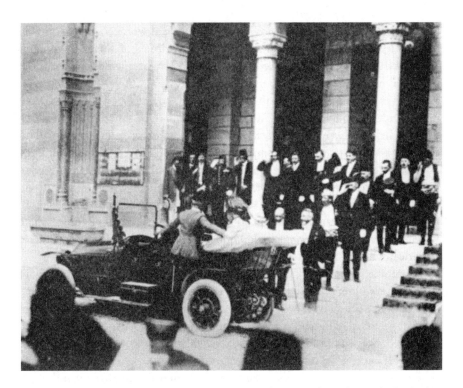

8. Archduke Franz Ferdinand and Duchess Sophie shortly before their assassination, Sarajevo.

ceremonial uniform, dark trousers with red stripes down the outside seams, blue double-breasted jacket with red piping, cuffs and high collar, ornately trimmed with gold braid and brass buttons, with a heavily plumed headdress and a sword at his side. He checks the curl of his handlebar moustache and it is quite as smart as it should be. She is in corseted white, with high neck, small belted waist and a flat-crowned hat with brim and veil, extravagantly trimmed with Vesuvius plume and a dark cockade to one side. Her hair is dressed in a soft swell, so that with the hat it forms an oval frame to her face. To either side a small guard of honour are dressed variously in Zouave trousers with striped ornamental sash and fez, in jellabas, in full-dress tie and tails and in modern dark sack suits.

Later that day the filming continues. After the first assassination attempt, the Archduke has exchanged his headdress for a plainer dark helmet with visor for his journey to the hospital to visit those that had been wounded earlier. After the fatal attack that follows, Count von Harrach, who was also in the vehicle, tries to wipe blood from the Archduke's lips, seizing him by his high coat collar to stop the Duke's head from falling forward. In the ensuing panic, attempts are made to uncover his chest in order to staunch the flow of blood, but eventually they realize they will have to cut the coat away. The Archduke was an immaculate dresser, so much so that he would have himself sewn into his many splendid uniforms in order to guarantee a perfect fit, with not a wrinkle to spoil the elegant line. By the time they had managed to get at the wound the Duke had died. Thus, this delay might be said to have been the catalyst for Austro-Hungary's declaration of war on Serbia. Dress – too great an attention to dress one might argue – was the cause of the First World War.

Weeks later the streets of Berlin were full of cheering crowds. Vienna at the outbreak of hostilities was resplendent with 'parades in the street, flags, ribbons and music burst forth everywhere [and] young recruits … marching triumphantly, their faces lighting up at the cheering'.[23] Piete Kuhr, in Schneidemühl, noticed military vehicles 'packed high with kitbags, underwear, trousers, jackets, caps, boots, ties and overcoats'.[24]

What did the crowds that gathered outside Buckingham Palace to cheer the King and Queen, or the troops that were amassing at Victoria Station feel but national pride? And their newly acquired uniforms, even their mock-ups of uniform of civilian suits with broom handles for rifles – how did these clothes enhance a sense of righteous moral purpose?[25]

Rupert Brooke, in a letter to John Drinkwater, cries, 'Come and die! It'll be great fun'.[26] War was meant to elevate mankind. Trivial concerns were to be set aside. In this heady maelstrom what did people choose to wear? Did their choices suddenly seem less or more significant? What clothing could sufficiently protect the participants of war, but also express a desire for sacrifice and for glory?

2 UNIFORM, CHIVALRY AND DOING ONE'S BIT

'It is really strange when we are naked; we are civilians again.'

Erich Maria Remarque, *All Quiet on the Western Front*

In the opening months of the First World War there was a rush to the colours: 250,000 men signed up in Britain alone in the first month. In Germany too, an atmosphere of confident victory meant that men were happy to volunteer. Twenty-five-year-old F. L. Cassel, of the 2nd Reserve German Army, went to a recruiting station with 'clean body, washed',[1] ready to be clothed identically to other men.

A uniform was something to anticipate with pride and could also allow entry into all manner of social milieu. An American serving in the Canadian military was impressed by the girls he saw on the streets of Paris, and found he held a surprising entrée to their acquaintance:

Uniform was my passport giving admission to cafes of dangerous repute and to refined homes alike.[2]

The detailed list of a German conscript's kit included 'grey uniform with red piping and bronze buttons, *Pickelhaube* [spiked helmet] with green cover, grey uniform cap, grey gloves ... two woollen jerseys, two pairs of underpants, four pairs of socks'. There is something exciting about new clothes, even when they are not of our choosing. To have them chosen for us can seem exhilarating. They can make us feel brand new.

Think of war and uniforms come to mind, though they are a relatively recent notion in modern warfare, post-seventeenth century for the main body of an army. Generals and admirals often adopted sumptuous and colourful regalia while their subordinates had to make do with whatever clothes they might happen to possess, a sash or armband distinguishing them from the opposing force. Moreover, officer ranks could be slow to adopt homogeneous clothing, too conscious of their status to wish to be so branded, as if in servants' livery. A Prussian nineteenth-century gorget say – a heart-shaped piece of metal worn to protect the throat and originating from medieval armoury – might offer good protection, but it was also valued because it retained something of its knightly past.

Uniforms can create a sense of communality and pride, but they can also feel demeaning to the wearer. It is sometimes argued that uniforms do away with economic and class discriminations, and yet we are all familiar with the ingenuity with which a school tie can be worn, high or low and with large or small knot, trainers that are state of the art or cut-price from a supermarket bin. All such distinctions can denote a subversive message, deliberately undercutting the cohesive intention of uniformed clothing, literally the 'uni'/ one form becoming many.

The very uniformity of uniform *en masse* can appear ridiculous and the individual may yearn to undermine it:

> One person dressed up, ready for serious publically authorized business, may be impressive, but a large group dressed all the same may be a little ludicrous because their appearance is so controlled and artificial.[3]

However, one might see uniform as not so much stifling the individual as allowing he or she scope to function as a soldier, nurse or ticket collector. John Harvey makes the point that uniform can act as a 'social force, they enrol us in armies'.[4] The Austrian novelist Hermann Broch suggests that such clothing's 'true function [is] to manifest and ordain order in the world … just as it conceals whatever in the human body is soft and flowing'.[5] This sense of repression might also trespass into a soldier's moral viewpoint, allowing him to act as otherwise, in home clothes, he might find difficult. When an act is committed by an individual under orders it is sanctioned as an act of the armed force and not of the individual; a person's uniform aids this sense of displaced responsibility. Even in hand-to-hand fighting with bayonets drawn, or ambushing sleeping troops for example, one might come to imagine one were killing not individuals in all their particularities, but an anonymous enemy, and *esprit de corps*, generated in part by uniform, might help to quash any sense of personal risk and guilt.

The way wars were fought was changing. New smokeless gunpowder,[6] barbed wire defences, grenades, the new armoured vehicles, gas attack, liquid fire and more accurate large and sniper small arms fire, meant that there was an increased need for both camouflage and protection. The physical demands of long-term entrenched fighting, risking not only military attack but the threat of water-borne disease and drowning, or troops embattled in icy conditions with little available shelter for example, made former standards of military sartorial verve dangerously out of place, and near impossible to maintain in the field.

Yet there remained times when practical concerns were overridden by the need to raise morale, and there was a need for clothing that suggested a noble past and was intended to strike fear into the opposing side. In a cavalry charge at Burkel in Flanders as late as 19 October 1918, many of the Belgian troops[7] wore traditional bearskins rather than metal helmets as they rode headlong into machine gun fire. Brandishing their sabres, some with lances held high for glory, swallow-tailed pennon flags fluttering, they must have seemed like medieval knights as the call went up the line, '*Hourra! ... En avant mes enfants ... pour le Roi!*' (Hurrah! ... Forward, my children ... for the King!).

Military uniforms had represented the height of male swagger during the Napoleonic Wars, worn with pride, 'showier and less comfortable than ever before or since'.[8] At the outset of the First World War uniforms still retained some of this splendour with brilliant colour and ornate decoration, with gilded braid Austrian knots, gilt buttons, vast Russian tasselled shoulder boards, dashing Hussars in looped *cadenette* plaits tossed back with fetching insolence from kohl-rimmed eyes, a lovelock tied with a ribbon like Charles I of England. There were silky curling Sikh moustaches and Zouave club-cut beards. Men with leg-defining, leg-lengthening stripes down the side of tightly tailored trews. These uniforms could make the most modestly built seem tall and muscular. They could transform a narrow-shouldered, soft-waisted silhouette and make it suddenly the ideal top-heavy, muscular, flab-free triangle. Ornate headgear was designed to suggest authority and threat, with Prussian Uhlans' rectangular-shaped helmets, spiked *Pickelhaube* helmets, top-heavy busbies resplendent with yellow and black plumes, tasselled fezzes and kepis and gorgeously wrapped turbans suggesting – to the Western eye – the exotic East.

The Russian military attempted to retain an old-fashioned formality to their version of khaki uniform, maintaining shoulder boards now of khaki braid, and adding to officers' and men's jackets a breastplate, or *plastron*, 'with buttons and collar attached, and false cuffs',[9] like an evening dicky, decency frill or lady's *chemisette*,[10] together with exaggeratedly tall, tapering caps. Despite these attempts to make new-style Russian uniform seem more romantic, Englishness was still generally considered suave. When the war broke out Russian officers took to wearing British loose service jackets, dubbing them 'Frenches', in honour of the British Commander-in-Chief, Sir John French.

Men of the Italian *Alpini* battalions, who fought in mountainous terrain against Austro-Hungarian *Kaiserjäger* and German *Alpenkorps*, were renowned for their marching songs, one such distinguishing them because of the ravens' feathers[11] on their caps: '*Sul cappello che noi portiamo ...*' (The cap that I wear ...) Officers wore white feathers on grey felt hats. This love of, literally, fine feathers, even in the direst conditions, is taken up again by Italian *Bersaglieri* (marksmen) regiments, light infantry troops wearing wide-brimmed hats, turned up to the side, adorned with prodigious curling *capercaillie* (wood grouse) feathers, which were later attached to the side of new steel combat helmets.

Since the Boer War, a much less practical uniform had been set aside for formal occasions alone, and the First World War necessitated even greater changes to service wear in the extreme conditions encountered. Yet men as we have seen were loath to abandon all to the meaner concerns of practicality in the field. Something of the old order – of the idea of noble display – remains in officers such as infantry Captain Hermann von Chappius in the Kaiser Franz Guard-Grenadiers, who according to his senior, Prince Kraft zu Hohenlobe-Ingelfingen, under heavy fire 'went fully erect in an elegant pace, as if he was leading the dance at court'. Chappius had been a leading dancer at the Potsdam court.[12]

The greatest diversity of elaborate uniform was to be found in Prussian regiments. Within the states of the German Empire the design of civilian and military uniform was relatively autonomous up to the First World War, and 'Bavaria, Saxony, and Wurttemberg guarded certain peculiarities',[13] such as wearing not only Empire cockades, but also those representing their own state, so that their helmets could seem as elaborate as a high fashion lady's concoction. There were also special badges and colourful sashes worn by the military of these different states, celebrating events before the period of German unification from 1866–71. To give up all such reference points would have represented a denial of their separate regimental histories.

For the Royal Welch Fusiliers, their history was tied up in both the archaic spelling of their name,[14] denoting their status as one of the oldest regiments of the British Army, and in a feature of dress, namely:

> A fan-like bunch of five black ribbons each 2" wide, 7.5" long, and ending in a dove-tail. The angle at which the fan must be spread has been exactly regulated by regimental convention. The flash is stitched to the back of the tunic collar, and only the Royal Welch are privileged to wear it.[15]

The 'flash', as it is termed, was sometimes worn at exaggerated lengths, flowing down the back like the pigtail, or queue, it had once adorned. In the First World War attempts were made to prevent the practice by the Army Council, who suggested it would be a target for snipers. Their commanding officer, Sir Luke O'Connor, parried that this was hardly a matter for concern, since there simply was no occasion, since the strategic withdrawal from Corunna in 1809 during the Peninsular Wars, that a Royal Welch Fusilier (RWF) had ever been known to show his back to the enemy. Although the matter was left unresolved, officers continued to sport the flash. The RWF dress uniform of scarlet jacket with navy blue facings was further embellished with a plume of white feathers, or hackle, on their fur caps, racoon-skin for the men, and bearskin for officers.

Those soldiers who attempted to maintain elements of their former colourful panache might risk drawing attention to themselves in the line, but the cut and dash, for example, of a turbaned and bearded Sikh battalion charge, on horseback and with lances raised, impressed their allies, and had the advantage of striking terror into the opposing side, partly on account of their very recklessness. An apocryphal story tells of Sikh soldiers returning to the trenches at nightfall and slowly unwinding their turbans before bed. As they did so, bullets that would otherwise surely have killed them, scatter to the ground. Thus these elegant men were considered lucky, defying death – and their company in battle might therefore be welcomed.

Those French army officers still in splendid red and blue at the outset of the war, their medals glinting in the light, sabres flashing, must have been a similarly fearsome sight, even if they were all too easily picked off by enemy fire. Gradually the bright colours of the French regiments, of which the red or '*garance* of the kepis and trousers [was] most noticeable',[16] were abandoned. At any rate, due to the sudden call on the army, one observer describes the majority of French troops at the beginning of the war as having to wear makeshift uniforms,

> dilapidated, scraped together uniforms. They wear those little caps, and dark blue coat, and red and blue trousers with two stripes running down the side … They mix the service and dress uniforms.[17]

French troops were at first given steel skullcaps, worn under their kepi caps, but the issue of the Adrian in the summer of 1915, the first steel combat helmet, provided better protection and was also adopted by Belgium, Italy, Serbia and Romania.[18] It had a raised ridge, or crest, along the top, front to back, like a French fire fighters' helmet, and was intended to deflect shrapnel and stop rain getting into an aeration valve at its apex. The Adrian was lightweight, with only a meagre leather and wool lining and weakened by its seams and rivets,[19] but at least went some way to protect against indirect fire. Following their lead, the British developed a stronger version, fashioned from a single sheet of metal and known as the Brodie, Shrapnel, Tommy hat or the Battle Bowler, and when adopted by American troops, the Doughboy helmet. The Brodie was at first, in October 1915, found too shallow and dangerously reflective, the rim too sharp and the lining too slippery to stay in place, but was improved in 1916 with a thicker, more cushioned leather liner and chin strap, and a matt-painted surface added, finished off with sand, sawdust or crushed cork. Although stronger, it still offered insufficient protection against a direct hit.

German forces were issued with the *Stahlhelm* (steel helmet), which had a slightly shallower crown and wider brim than the Brodie, but was also lined for greater comfort and stability, and again held in place with a chinstrap of leather: medieval *sallet* to Allied *chapel-de-fer* perhaps. *Stahlhelmes* were fashioned from a stronger, thicker layer of steel than either types of Allied helmet, but they also had to be adapted, as they covered the ears too closely, making hearing difficult, resulting in the outward curving design retained into the Second World War. Despite these innovations, along with busbies, shakos and shapkas, *Pickelhauben* were still being worn by many soldiers right up until the armistice in November 1918.[20]

In Serbia the *ajkaca* cap, worn in the eighteenth century by uniformed river fleet men, was fashioned from thickened boiled wool in the shape of a pillbox, with a crease down the centre formed in a V-shaped seam and with a pair of earflaps attached. Due to an accidental over-ordering, they went into service as general army headgear early in the twentieth century, and were worn by Persian military forces. In the First World War these were worn by all ranks, officers' caps having additional rigid peaks attached, though a simpler conical shepherd's cap, or *ubura*, was also worn. Both caps were adopted as national costume. The *ajkaca* was a distinctive item of dress for Yugoslav royalist resistance fighters in the Second World War and worn by Bosnian Serb military commanders in the Bosnian War of the early 1990s – a small piece of felt taking on a powerful sense of national significance. Another example of an accidental uniform choice concerns British and Canadian 'Air Force' blue. Large quantities of light blue cloth were ordered by the Tsarist army, but lay unwanted after the October Revolution of 1918. In 1920, when the RCAF and RAF were formed, this leftover cloth was adopted and continues to be worn today, the term 'air force blue' used widely for this particular shade.

A hat, of course, is an easily recognizable symbol of identity. The Ottoman *Kabalak* cap was still worn, the most common form being made up of bands of khaki cloth wrapped round a wicker frame, like an upturned flowerpot.[21] For the Cossacks, the Astrakhan cap was the defining item of clothing for its various corps, in slightly different styles, all made of fleece, sometimes with distinctive coloured felt tops. The Tsar's personal escort, the *Konvoi*, were the most elaborately uniformed Cossacks, wearing brilliant scarlet coats and with their caps emblazoned with red crowns. The Kaiser resisted the idea of less colourful uniforms, though the delay in supply of both steel helmets and field grey uniforms was for economic rather than sartorial reasons. In Germany, though ranks were officially allocated new uniforms from 1907 (and the more reluctant officers from 1910), substantial stocks of blue material meant that the German army was still being issued the older-style uniforms well into the war.

In *All Quiet on the Western Front*, the protagonist's uniform signifies his identity as a soldier. He has become part of a united force, protected from the world at large, the 'textile armor' imposing an unassailable military posture 'to produce the illusion of a collective masculinization'.[22] I would argue that this is not so much an illusion, for to become masculine in this context involves asserting a belief in one's own strength and authority, and relies upon how one is seen by one's fellows, by civilians and ultimately by the enemy. The clothed outer is thus essential in creating the soldier.

So, uniforms can separate those who fight from civilians. They legitimate authority and the rule of force. To wear a uniform is to offer oneself up to the opposing side in a conflict, and as a particular group, regiment or nationality within an army, hence the phrase 'to declare one's colours'. A certain rivalry between factions fighting on the same side could boost morale, so that the tribulations of warfare might seem more like sport. Scottish Highland regiments earned a reputation for ruthlessness so that the mere sight of their kilts could strike fear into the enemy and dare those fighting alongside to be as fearless. On the one hand, the kilt one might contend was an ideal garment, its eight and a quarter yards of pleated wool under a khaki apron keeping the men warm, yet cool in summer, a group of Australian soldiers attempting to follow suit in Gallipoli:

> most of us have cut down our infantry trews at the knees. As my knicks are fairly baggy I can quite realize what it feels like to wear kilts.[23]

On the other hand, the kilt 'was in many ways a handicap in trench warfare, the quantity of cloth difficult to dry out in wet conditions and finally had to be abandoned when it was realized that mustard gas tended to burn the sweatier parts of the body, with disastrous consequences'.[24] The Scottish regiments had 12 different cut-away styles of jacket, to allow for the sporran. Spats had also to be abandoned for practical reasons.

Even the smallest items of dress could be a liability, when on a reconnaissance mission close to the German trenches one such almost gives a group of men away:

> Going out we had to get under our barbed wire and do it on your back, and the button of my [tunic] caught and it rang out like the bells of St Paul's, but it was alright.[25]

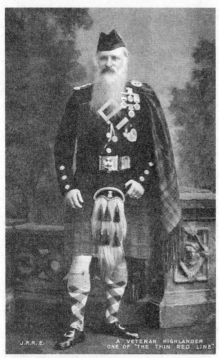

J.R.R.E.

A VETERAN HIGHLANDER
ONE OF "THE THIN RED LINE"

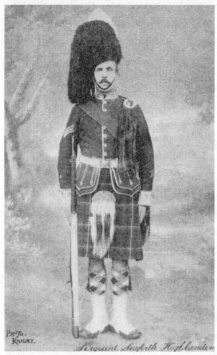

Photo.
Knight.

Sergeant Seaforth Highlander

9. The Scottish kilt worn with pride.

Inversely buttons were the solution to the problem many British troops encountered in muddy terrain, when their coats could become saturated and heavy:

> I had cut my greatcoat at the bottom because it was soaked in mud and hard ... and I cut it off. That was a crime ... interfering with military property.[26]

This was a punishable offence, and eventually a system of tabs and buttons was developed, so that in wet weather the coat could be rolled up and buttoned out of the way.

The Twentieth-Century Uniform

When modern firepower allowed much fighting to be conducted at a distance it followed that uniforms were less necessary to distinguish soldiers from the opposing force, yet differentiations, as I have suggested, remained, 'to reflect the military traditions of armies rather than to distinguish the force from other armies, and even less to distinguish it from the civilian population'.[27]

The difficulty of the transfer from conspicuous to more practical uniform in colour and design should not be understated. In the new fighting conditions a change in men's attitudes to themselves as soldiers came about. If you could kill and maim at a distance, then you could avoid one-to-one contact, at least in theory. The fighting men of the First World War were at the cusp of this changeover. The extent to which old sartorial values were clung to, and conversely how quickly armies were to take advantage of a certain depersonalizing distance from the enemy, was to have a telling effect on armies' fighting proficiency.

If uniforms suggest allegiance, then in contrast, guerrilla warfare, which by definition avoids identifying clothing, was considered to be sly and dishonourable. Peter Englund discusses how guerrilla tactics were viewed as uncivilized in the First World War and led to acts of bloody reprisal against civilians thought to be responsible for atrocities, both in Belgium and in Serbia at the beginning of the conflict.[28] However, espionage, which also involves concealing one's loyalties, was often seen as particularly brave, perhaps on account of the severe measures a spy can expect if detected. Enemy spies or enemy subterfuge in general, was of course less admired.

A lack of uniform can seem to imply guilt. Mata Hari, the alleged German spy, is described at her execution by firing squad as brazenly wearing 'a neat Amazonian tailored suit, especially made for the occasion, and a pair of new white gloves'.[29] Her fashionable civilian clothing appeared to *The New Yorker* magazine (1934) to imply that there was something unseemly, and possibly wasteful, in donning *new* gloves when one was about to die. Pat Shipman argues that Mata Hari had little choice in the matter, and that the only clean clothes made available to her were the said suit and tricorn hat. This hat was then claimed to have 'mocked the military establishment', even though it was in fact provided by the French authorities.[30] It is probable that they wished her clothing to suggest something of her sexually voracious and fashion-conscious past, and thus a character easily led and morally shallow.

Uniforms could be used to deliberately misinform. Sister Cecile, a British nun in a community near Antwerp under German occupation, testily reports in her diary in November 1915 when a German aircrew crashes nearby:

> A flying machine came down quite close to the Convent; they tried to go up again, but failed, and two men had to be extricated from under the machine. Belges applauded. The [German] officers then put on English uniforms and were photographed for the German papers. This is always done, we hear!!![31]

Uniform is being used here for the purposes of propaganda, insinuating that it is the enemy alone whose aircraft crash.

A uniform can transform how the wearer is treated. In 1906 in Köpenick, east of Berlin, a down-and-out Friedrich Wilhelm Voigt had only to assume an officer's uniform in order to be treated as a respected member of the community, able to arrest the town treasurer and mayor and 'confiscate' a large sum of money in the name of the Kaiser. What has been termed the 'Prussian Cult of the Uniform', denoting how serving in the military is a means of gaining respect and trust, allows Voigt to commandeer a troop of soldiers. In a play based on his life[32] Voigt glimpses himself in a mirror in his adopted uniform, and he roars with laughter at the ridiculous sight – at the ability mere clothing has to change how a man is seen.

When Vera Brittain, working as a Voluntary Aid Detachment (VAD) nurse in 1915, first sees her fiancé Roland Leighton dressed for war, she finds that both the virile role he now inhabits, and her awareness of it, diminishes her as a woman in her civilian fripperies:

> his uniform and little moustache had changed him from a boy into a man, and one so large and powerful that even in the splendour of the rose-trimmed hat and new squirrel coat ... I felt like a midget beside him.[33]

A young Central Powers' recruit, Adolf Hitler, took pride in his new field grey uniform, and it is curious to see how strong a resemblance it bore to the clothing he later wore as *Führer*. Unlike many of his senior command, who had a taste for excess, Hitler chose to dress simply, his earlier military moustache became smaller, wearing a white shirt, black tie, black trousers and a double-breasted grey jacket with the revers turned back. His only decoration was a gold Nazi Party badge, a black wound badge, and his Iron Cross 1st Class. The image he cuts is deliberately unassuming:

> He needed a 'uniform' worn by no one else, and he chose one with an unsuspected taste for understatement.[34]

It was a uniform that deliberately harked back to the First World War and associated him with the ordinary foot soldier of that time.

Our contemporary response to the notion of uniform can be one of embarrassment. It can seem war mongering to feel moved by the sight of soldiers in medals and military finery. In 1914, a stirring of pride for men kitted out for war – in however stopgap a manner – would have been a far more common response. For the first wave of troops that faced the frontline trenches, their expectations of brief battle fought like the heroes they had read about as boys were destroyed by the experience of a slow war of attrition, where previous elements of military splendour were gradually abandoned.

Practical Solutions

Some aspects of traditional uniform worn on both sides were less sumptuous. Leg wraps had been a means of the poor keeping warm in winter since early history, and are a feature of Russian and Greek folk and national dress, for example. Essentially they did not require any sewing, were easily made from old clothes or sacking and could be used to cover the foot as well, in lieu of expensive footwear – hence the term 'toe rag' as an expression of contempt. Canvas field grey, grey blue and khaki puttees were their sturdier progeny, a name derived from the Hindu word for bandage, *patti*, and first used by the British Army in the Himalayas as a substitute for leather anklets or gaiters.

Men were often late for roll call simply because of the difficulty of putting on their puttees and they were hard to keep in place without them becoming too tight and therefore uncomfortable, or too loose and falling down:

> The rolling of puttees was a mystery ... The rolls opened like the gills of fishes; they were too thick round the ankle or too tight round the calf.[35]

Although they were intended to keep the water and mud out and protect the feet, in wet conditions they could shrink, impeding the circulation to the

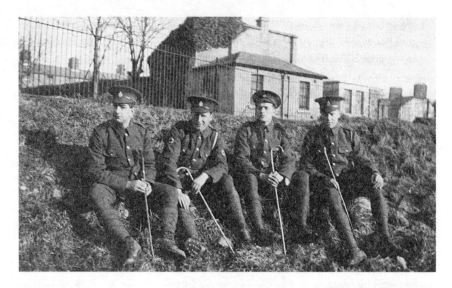

10. Soldiers serving in Limerick, Ireland and in the Middle East, 1914-16.

foot, and greatly exacerbating conditions such as trench foot and frostbite. However, they were regularly used in the field as tourniquets, and could be taken from a severed leg, say, and turned with a length of shell fragment to stop the flow of blood.

On the Western Front, from the North Sea along the shifting lines to the Swiss frontier with France, armies were entrenched throughout the course of the war. In wet weather mud filled these trenches and became like Portland cement, getting into every crevice. A German recruit writes in his diary of a freezing night on 12 December 1915 with 'our boots full of the wet mud-soup'.[36] The same young soldier describes the pantomime of marching in muddy conditions:

> Those who had gum-boots on kept catching hold of the loops on each side of the boot that had to make a step forward and hauling it out of the mud. In spite of this, somebody got stuck every moment, and then the whole file was held up. Generally the front and rear man of the one who had got stuck seized his foot and dragged it out. We often sank over our knees in the morass. Some men had their boots pulled right off and stood in their stockings, or even bare-foot, pressing themselves against the wall to let others pass, before trying to retrieve them.[37]

In similar vein, the British private, Harold Hayward, describes his experience of muddy conditions in October 1915:

> We put our braces through the loops of the gum-boots … and being rubber gum-boots, and there was mud … [it] acted like a sucker and you couldn't move, couldn't pull your foot out.[38]

A Salvation Army officer, ministering to the British and American troops in France in 1915, comments that even if a soldier wore hip-length boots 'he must take them off every little while and empty the mud out, which somehow manages to get into even them'.[39]

New boots could be a considerable problem. Marching with heavy packs on their backs, new reservists in 1914 were provided with

> 'ammos' (that's the old army word for boots) and they were very heavy. Before the war we were able to break them in, but they didn't get the time. They were put straight out to march 150, 160 miles with only a very few rests and if they did get those boots off they didn't get them back on again, consequently their feet were bleeding.[40]

A sergeant forced to march in new boots in April of 1915 near Ypres, comments that a 'good many Belgian women came out of their cottages and bathed our feet and bandaged them up as we sat by the road'.[41]

The British Army issued whale oil for troops to rub into their feet to avoid foot complaints, which might otherwise lead to gangrene and amputation. Women on both sides of the conflict were encouraged to knit warm socks for their soldiers, which was just as well, since standard British[42] and German uniform supplies sometimes included only one spare pair and it was essential that troops' feet were in reasonable condition if the were to be kept mobile.

The Officer Class and Making Do

Uniform is intended to be smart, to instil a sense of discipline. Certainly many officers saw it as a mark of their gentlemanly status to have their uniforms bespoke, rather than risk army issue. Across the board officers had their uniforms tailor-made.[43] There were logistical problems in relying on military issue, a German doctor bound for East Prussia and later Gallipoli, expressing his impatience:

> At the officers' club I was carefully measured for a uniform, but when I asked when I could have the first fitting I was told 'in six weeks'. That long I could not wait. A private tailor accomplished everything needed, faultlessly, within 48 hours.[44]

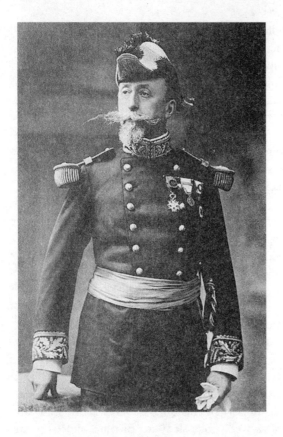

11. High-ranking French officer,
Étienne de Villaret, 1912.

In the British Army, the trench coat was permitted, as with the Winter Warm short coat, for officers and warrant officers Class I alone, as an optional item of dress, and many variations were made. Burberry had developed gabardine cloth and lighter-weight waterproofed poplin for raincoats. It was adapted for wartime conditions with added epaulettes and D rings, and became a popular alternative to the heavy and easily sodden greatcoat. It had a waterproof silk interlining and a removable, heavy wool button-in lining for cold weather, the fashion magazine *Vanity Fair* advising the well-dressed man that:

> Such a coat will afford complete protection, even under the most trying conditions of trench or open field.[45]

Female versions of the trench coat were made in a wider variety of fabrics for uniformed auxiliary units, one such version having an optional additional fleece lining, in a 'tan cravenetted serge, interlined with flannel and lined with serge'.[46]

German army trench coats were made along very similar lines to the Burberry, but in field grey and introduced later in the war for officers of means. Some British officers wore khaki shirts of a subtly deeper khaki than their men's mass-produced ones. In the novel *Regeneration*, Prior, who is of a lower class background, describes how this affected other officers' attitudes towards him in training:

> It's made perfectly clear when you arrive that some people are more welcome than others. It helps if you've been to the right school. It helps if you hunt, it helps if your shirts are the right colour. Which is a *deep* shade of khaki, by the way.[47]

In the novel *Greenmantle*, Richard Hannay is advised by a fellow officer to, 'Try my tailor ... He's got a very nice taste in red tabs. You can use my name'.[48] He is being offered access to a tailor who, by implication, cannot be got merely by money. Such an introduction, not available to all comers, is a crucial distinguishing feature of class advantage here.

Officers, intending to cut a dash, and of sufficient means, might have been able to kit themselves out at their tailors, but such distinctions went against the general ethos of unifying the lower and officer ranks. A sergeant might decide that he would look more the part when 'tunic and trousers had been taken in tighter than regulation fit by the depôt tailor',[49] yet even for a well-to-do officer, the expense could be prohibitive. Once the nature of the combat and its heavy impact on their clothes had been experienced, many resorted to more standard-issue suppliers, there being few opportunities for swank in the field. An American pilot who had volunteered and trained with a French *escadrille* (air squadron) writes to his mother about the expense of keeping his uniform in good order when what had been issued wore out:

> we live expensively, seven and eight course meals, and your valet and crew of mechanicians eat into that old check ... I also ruined a nearly new $56 uniform in that smash in July, oil, rips and tears it was useless.[50]

Lower ranks' new uniforms were often ill fitting due to the logistical problem of matching individual men with the sizes available. Depending upon the assiduity of the commanding officer, or sheer luck, some regiments faired better than others, according to one recruit in training near Bristol:

> I think we had two sets, one for special purposes and one for when we were out practicing field fighting because of lying down on the ground ... another outfit for walking out ... we certainly got ours long before others ... they must have got in very early with their order.[51]

As the need for Earl Kitchener's army of volunteers increased, uniform shortages meant that men were forced to train in their own clothing and footwear, with perhaps just a regimental badge sewn onto their sleeve. In some cases Boer War red jackets were issued, and in others a temporary uniform was supplied of cheap blue cloth, which became known as Kitchener's blue:

> wearing out their own shoe leather for want of army boots, patching, darning
> and inexpertly cobbling together holes that inevitably appeared in elbows and
> knees of suits that had never been intended for wear.

Even when the manufacturers managed to meet the demand and khaki service uniform was made available at last, the men posing for photographs often 'still had no belt or cap, for the equipment arrived in dribs and drabs'.[52]

During training, a corporal recalls one volunteer suffering the ignominy of having to remain in his own suit, since his unusually stocky yet short-legged frame had so far proved impossible to clothe:

> Poor old Pendry had to parade every day in a black suit and bowler hat.[53]

Yet while the war was still young and recruits had hopes of it being over by the first Christmas, ill-fitting uniforms were met with good humour:

> Goodness what a fit, but don't shoot the tailor, he's doing his best. It was take it
> or leave it … we had a general swop round with caps and tunics, resulting in a
> much more presentable appearance.[54]

In the field, the escalating conflict required more and more men, and given the conditions, uniforms were often worn to shreds before they could be replaced. As early as 1915, an officer comments when British troops strip off for a rare hot bath that 'many of their clothes are in rags, but [they] cannot be replaced, we are told, until they get much worse'.[55]

After a group of soldiers have taken a bath at a delousing station in Poperinghe Flanders, their underwear is returned fumigated, but not necessarily to the right men:

> If you were lucky you got some that nearly fitted you, but, of course, I was the
> wrong size for that and it would always happen to me that I got huge underwear.
> They were all Long Johns in those days, and by the time I'd done them up they
> were right around my chest, and I'd also have to take about three folds in the
> bottom of the legs. That would be topped with a vest hanging down to my knees.
> On the other hand, a fellow who was a six-footer would be issued with a set so

small that he could hardly get into it at all, so we had to swop around as best we could.[56]

Piete Kuhr, the young German girl, mentions German soldiers returning from the Eastern Front in May 1915, 'their uniforms ... dirty and torn'. Through the course of her diary she gradually brings together all the elements of a worn out uniform, so that one day she will have a costume capable of representing an everyman, a puppet soldier, for a dance she intends to perform herself, entitled *The Dead Soldier.*

> I made up a life-size long figure – head, chest, legs, everything, and covered it with a black coach-rug just as if this was plainly supported by the body underneath it. Then I placed Uncle Bruno's old army boots next to each other in military fashion and sticking out from under the cloth ... I placed on the dented, flat, steel helmet.[57]

When later her brother arrives home at the end of the war, she immediately recognizes that his torn and dishevelled uniform will be perfect to complete her outfit:

> His uniform was open over his shirt, the buttons had been torn off taking bits of cloth with them, the shoulder-strips had likewise been torn off, his collar was dangling halfway down, and he had neither sword belt nor forage cap ... I held the uniform tight against me with both arms, sobbing bitterly – the poor, poor, German field uniform.[58]

In POW camps difficulties maintaining uniform were even more extreme. Anything that could be recycled was put to use in a Bavarian jail housing a variety of different nationalities, including 'a gigantic chasseur d'Afrique' making a cap out of a red trouser leg and a dragoon fashioning a police cap out of the same stuff.[59] Often Russians suffered particularly harsh treatment in enemy hands, a British POW reporting seeing a cattle truck of prisoners being taken to dig German trenches, 'who were hardly alive, smelt, full of lice ... a few tattered clothes on them ... [a] most pathetic sight'.[60] However, when Russians join a group of French prisoners, they swap clothing, as much for the enjoyment of dressing up as for their practical needs:

> kepi for toque, fatigue cap for its Russian equivalent. After a few days the Russian buttons stamped with the two-headed eagle had found their way on to our coats, while the French grenade buttons were displayed upon the huge Russian earth-coloured cloaks. Tartar feet were encased in French army shoes; while red

trousers were tucked into the supple boots of Ukraine leather. Early Christian communism prevailed. Everyone dressed as he fancied, mixing the uniforms of the two armies. For an entire week the height of fashion in numbers 44 and 46 [cells], aristocratic regions, was to walk out in *moujiks* [embroidered] blouses.[61]

From a broader perspective, recycling became essential to support the war effort on all sides (discussed further in Chapter 4). In France alone, 287,000 skilled men were brought back from active service to work in salvage and recycling.[62] For the British during the Somme:

> Clothing was cleaned and repaired, or, if beyond redemption, sent back ... as rags. Steel helmets were cleaned and relined if they were whole, or, if too battered and holed, were sold as scrap iron after the chin straps had been removed for sale as old leather ... Webbing equipment was dry-cleaned on motor-driven brushes, darned and repaired by local labour, or, if beyond repair, had their metal fittings removed and were sent back ... as cotton rags ... [F]ish oil [was] used to restore old boots, even boots whose useful life was at an obvious end had their studs removed for scrap metal before they were abandoned.[63]

Friendship and Dress

In *All Quiet on the Western Front*, Paul Bäumer talks of 'surrendering our individual personalities' in training, yet it is the nuance of the friendships within his squad that are central to the plot. His close friend Müller longs for more comfortable boots, as those issued had cardboard soles that could not withstand wet weather.[64] Inheriting superior boots from a dead comrade, in his last dying moments Bäumer bequeaths them to Müller, and they seem to embody that friendship.[65] Away from family and facing danger, the bonds that grew up between soldier and soldier helped sustain a fighting force, and it was often in small matters of sharing – of clothing, of precious soap, cigarettes and so on – that built up trust and mutual reliance. In the German lines in Gallipoli, a doctor notices how the men's affection for their young lieutenant is expressed through the care they take over his clothing, so that he will not be ashamed to be seen on leave:

> I saw how a company was busy trying with all the tricks to clean up the war-soiled uniform.[66]

A soldier working in the British Army Service Corps, carrying up replacement uniform and boots into the lines in Gallipoli, eschews time away in relative comfort to recuperate from dysentery, preferring to return to his fly-ridden dugout, to the soldier he worked with, 'to my pal'.[67]

***

The kinds of impression a soldier made affected not only his readiness for battle, but might also have a bearing on his personal attractions. For example, one young woman arriving in France from America in 1914, when the switch to khaki had not been completed, describes the French soldiers as looking messy:

> Their gaudy uniforms remind me of Wallace Irwin's pun on French trousers: Toulon, Toulouse and too baggy.

She is more impressed with the English troops she encounters, 'trimly dressed in khaki. Nice clean-looking fellows',[68] though in fact many British soldiers would also have still been in makeshift uniform.

The first trickle of American troops arriving in France in 1916 were similarly poorly kitted out, uniformed in a mock-khaki cotton material, 'badly fitting, very ordinary, and I regret to say it, dirty'.[69] America's sudden involvement in the war, after the German attack on its Atlantic shipping, meant that supplies including clothing were insufficient to meet the quantities required. General Pershing was unwilling to adopt European Allied uniforms, in order to preserve the independent identity of his countrymen; he did not want them used merely to replace other armies' vacancies, piecemeal.

By the following year there had been sufficient time to train and uniform new recruits, so that the American Expeditionary Force *en masse* made a rather different impression 'trim in new khaki, the new battle-caps perched jauntily'.[70] However, it should be remembered that the uniforms we might see today housed in a museum are unlikely to be those that were worn in the field:

> Most of the surviving examples are 'walking out' uniforms, never worn except for the return home. Other uniforms ... were changed, repaired, deloused, reissued or sent to the salvage heap.[71]

Once they had become embroiled in the conflict the difficulties that the other forces had encountered, of extreme conditions and problems in maintaining supplies similarly affected American volunteers. Allen Peck, writes home as late as 1917 about being measured for his pilot's uniform, and of being uncertain 'when I will get it ... am drilling etc. in that brown suit'.[72]

Use of aeroplanes in military combat was at its naissance and first used only for reconnaissance flights. German Fokkers and French and British craft were of fragile construction with mainly wooden frames covered in a skin of fabric. Decisions had to be made about appropriate clothing. At first aviators tended to wear their previous regimental uniforms, gradually making adaptations to suit their needs. They wore items such as leather helmets with ear flaps attached, goggles and fur-lined gloves, essential accoutrements when cockpits were open to the elements, and sometimes fleece-lined leather double-breasted reefer jackets, with deep revers and collars that could be turned up against foul weather.

Whereas the British Royal Flying Corps are pictured in long leather coats at the beginning of the war,[73] in 1917 American pilots were issued with short flying jackets, zipped and fitted with wind flaps and a collar that could be worn high to the chin. As with field trench coats, open pocket slits allowed access to the jacket beneath, which meant solo flyers could reach into the pockets of their service tunics. As attempts were made to design uniforms specifically for pilots, it is apparent that these men wanted more from a uniform than merely practical features. The role of pilot was a respected one. They were seen as daredevils of the sky, and their clothing needed not only to keep them warm and safe but also to live up to a mythical image that increased their status.

Given the risks they ran, pilots' clothing had both to dignify their new role as warriors in a new dimension, but also had to allow for a degree of diversity. These were individuals, acting solo for a common cause. Looking at German pilots at the time it is difficult to find any two dressed alike. Notably breeches were designed as if for horseback, with leather reinforcements on the inside leg and often black leather riding boots,[74] as if the former swagger of the noble horseman has been transposed to the air. For these first flyers and the overwhelming risks they ran, with no parachutes and planes that were highly flammable due to the 'dope' that was used to strengthen the canvas skin, these makeshift adaptations have had a lasting effect on the resonance of leather and fur, breeches and high fitted boots.

Given the nature of the high risk, one-to-one combat that ensued – after it became possible to mount a machine gun on board, synchronizing its fire with the propeller – then it is not surprising that these first flying aces entered the realm of the hero. This accounts I think for a certain nonchalance in their uniform style, a freedom from the severe restrictions of group orders, wearing their loosely tied silk scarves, goggles pushed back like the dark glasses of a film star. They are pictured with cigarette in hand, smiling, twirling a moustache, hands in pockets, devil-may-care.

Chivalrous Combat

What effect did the dulling down of uniform have on a sense of war as glorious chivalric adventure? Lord Wolseley in 1889, comments on the advantages of theatrical, impractical clothing, 'strange to say, [soldiers] like very tightly fitting coats and trousers, to swagger about in with their sweethearts ... This applies to all ranks',[75] and Remarque draws a direct comparison:

> The steel-helmeted cavalrymen look like knights in armour from a bygone age
> – somehow it is moving and beautiful.[76]

The 'holy war' of the Allies, the righteous crusade of the Central Powers, both called on a medieval masculine ideal of a man as knight in shining armour, even if the reality lay in armies in field grey, blue grey, dull green and khaki, often ill equipped and shabby. Here was little of the imagined audacity of the nineteenth-century soldier. Yet there is perhaps something of chivalric glamour in accounts of soldiers being seen off on board ships or at railway stations. Vera Brittain recalls taking leave of Roland Leighton, where gloves are at first a physical material barrier and their removal an emotional connection:

> He took my hand and kissed it again as he did in the train once before – but this
> time there was no glove upon it.[77]

In poetry[78] this association between war and its chivalric connotations is played out. The suggestion of the knightly duty to protect women had great romantic and political potential, when from both sides of the conflict damsels might be in need of protection from the lascivious Serb or barbaric Bulgarian. Though some women did seek to fight, for many the war thrust them into an all too familiar supportive role, even if it could at times be coloured by resentment:

> Oh it's you that have the luck, out there in blood and muck:
> ... In a trench you are sitting, while I am knitting
> A hopeless sock, that never gets done.[79]

This war was to draw in most of the established armies of the developed world, engaging colonial forces, so that the struggle to cohere as two distinct sides, and still maintain some sense of their individual allegiances and history, in part relied on the uniforms that were adopted. The assumption of uniform was a means of transforming the individual into that 'person associated with the values [war] represents, and thus [she or he] increases in courage, obedience, loyalty and intellect by the act of putting on ... livery'.[80]

When Norman Stone describes the occasion of the Treaty of Brest-Litovsk in 1917 between the Bolsheviks and Germany, he looks to the dress of the participants to uncover the snobberies and tensions that in part motivated their decisions. Referring to this first filming of a diplomatic treaty, Prince Leopold of Bavaria holds court in Field Marshal's uniform. The Central European aristocrats lack the splendour of military uniform, but they are confident in their gravitas 'leaning back patronizingly in black ties'.[81]

Photographs of sweetheart or wife, a present of a homemade vest or comforter sent into the lines increased a sense of allegiance (as detailed in Chapter 4) what one young German describes as representing 'what Germany has done for us'.[82] These precious parcels take on something of the potency of a medieval lady's favour. In this tournament of war, just as in courtly custom a champion might accept a token from his lady, a veil, ribbon or piece of jewellery, gifts from home could shore up courage, making it a point of honour to fight on. Siegfried Sassoon cuts through this pretty parallel in a bitter complaint against a certain female response to war, which coyly delights in wounds 'in a mentionable place':

you believe / That chivalry redeems the world's disgrace.[83]

Gifts could be lucky, the pilot Allen Peck asking for a stuffed, black toy cat to hang on wires on the front of his plane[84] 'to aid my friend Dame Fortune in keeping her relative Miss Fortune from climbing onto my plane', and mentions other flyers' charms. 'I have seen elephants, lions, chickens and nearly everything.' He also begs a stocking cap to protect him from wind chill. Silk stockings were sometimes worn over the entire face and were also thought, erroneously, to offer some protection from fire.

In courtly love it was part of a lady's duty to prepare her knight for battle by sewing his shirts or embroidering his armorial ensign. The distance these separate roles enforced, of formal exchange of symbolic gift and domestic provision, fed into ideas of the honourable gentleman whose role was to protect. This in turn affected underlying male attitudes to the First World War, imbuing them with a sense of manly duty. Such ideals made it possible for fighting men to keep fighting, as a matter of honour, even when they had cause to doubt the righteous purpose of the war.

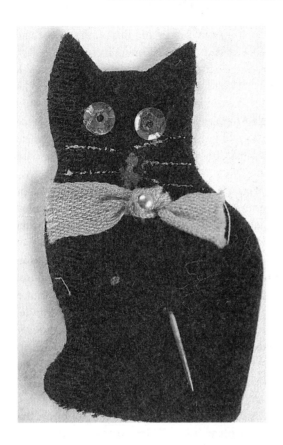

12. A black felt cat used as a lucky charm.

Soldiers of Colour

African American and West Indians volunteering to fight in the war found that they were at first used as a brute labour force, digging trenches, clearing mines, repairing roads and recovering bodies from no-man's-land, like the Chinese, Indian and Burmese labour forces, and were also used as stevedores at Brest and other ports. Many African Americans were given old Civil War uniforms to wear in training and 'literacy tests were used to justify assigning blacks to labor units'.[85] The unwillingness on the part of the American government to trust these men on the frontline, to see them armed and uniformed on a par with white soldiers, meant that many opted to transfer to the 16th French Division where they were allowed to fight. They wore American khaki standard issue uniform, but with French rifles, gas masks and Adrian helmets. With something to prove, these men quickly gained a reputation for fighting prowess, yet it is a telling irony of dress that they were depicted wearing American Brodie helmets, an honour they did not receive until the last months of the war. Walter Dean Myers and Bill Miles suggest that the success of these black soldiers, and the military honours they received, were in part responsible for an outbreak of race violence and lynchings in post-war America:

> Some of them were veterans of the war still in their uniforms. There were so many deaths and so much bloodshed during the hot months of 1919 that it was called Red Summer.[86]

Troops drawn from colonial Africa found themselves kitted out in Western-style clothing, and if these uniforms were not returned, they often became high-status garb post-war. Officials and missionaries alike tried to inhibit the custom of the former soldiers continuing to war combat gear. They attempted to impose a new mode of 'African' dress instead, much like that worn by village natives in Tarzan films, of simple 'modest' shifts tied with a sash, sometimes one-shouldered in a nod to animal skin traditional garb. In post-war Western Africa, Winston Churchill missed the sartorial cultural compliment when he railed against tribal leaders for cherishing 'any old cast-off khaki jacket or tattered pair of trousers'.[87] Their uniforms had become honorary clothing, adopted as 'symbols of modernity and power', as had often been the practice regarding artefacts from previous invasions of their culture.

The French were prepared to incorporate colonial troops into their army, unlike the Belgians and British who preferred to use 'ethnic' labourers for ancillary duties rather than as a fighting force. There was a fear that, like the perceived threat from black Americans, such trained troops might learn too much, both in terms of weaponry and confidence in relation to those they should view as superior, and therefore prove a threat to the authority of their masters after the war. In such non-combative roles, what they wore was considered of less importance. These men, often accustomed to a warm, predominantly dry climate, had to manage with whatever they could find to protect them from the cold and damp, since their uniforms consisted of what had been rejected as sub-standard, or too damaged for use by other troops. Clothing that mixes facets of military with civilian gear can make one and the other lose ground, as with Chinese dock workers in France wearing a random assortment of clothing, 'ladies' blouses, black satin trousers, old coats, soldiers' tunics – anything'.[88]

These difficulties only apply to Allied colonial troops on the Western Front, since it proved impossible for Central Powers to ship German colonial troops into Europe on account of the British naval blockade.

Colonial expansion meant that some indigenous forces had already received military training, and were brought into the war with some aspects of tribal and ethnic clothing already part of their uniforms. The North African *Tirailleurs* of the French army, for example, wore Zouave-style voluminous trousers, broad sashes and red fezzes, the *Spahis* more elaborate still with flowing white *burnous* robes with a red cloak (Moroccan regiments wearing blue) with short red jackets, sky blue waistcoats and topped off with a high white Arab headdress. The *Zouaves*, a light infantry corps drawn from French settlers in North Africa, wore short, open-fronted jackets and baggy trousers with sashes, along with a range of exotic headgear of fezzes, tasselled caps or *tarbouches* and turbans. Like Scottish and Sikh regiments, something of the verve of their outfits lent them an air of recklessness, the French vernacular *faire le Zouave* meaning to behave in a wild manner. Something of this allure survived even after the first months of the war, even when they began to be kitted out in khaki service dress and steel helmets.

While both the Belgian and British allowed non-Europeans to rise only to the rank of sergeant, the French allowed them to become officers, which meant they were better able to retain some aspects of their former uniform. The brimless *tarbouches* were sometimes worn into battle, even though strictly speaking this was against regulations, with only turbans being permitted for religious reasons. The fez had already filtered into European use, with Bosnian infantry regiments, for example, wearing them throughout the war. Men in the line wore muted brown fezzes with a long black wool tassel worn to the rear, though officers wore the Austrian military cap, unless they were Muslim.

In contrast to the *Tirailleurs*, the French Foreign Legion, who were formed from volunteers of many non-French nationalities including American and European recruits, had uniforms designed for the North African sun, but with less of an oriental appearance. The trousers were less baggy and the dark blue tunics with red collars and kepi caps with round flat tops, with a horizontal peak piped and banded with blue, bear a far closer resemblance to standard French early twentieth-century uniform. They did, however, like the *Zouaves*, wear the Beau Geste wide white linen trousers in summer, tucked into leather leggings. Nevertheless, fighting on the Western Front, they soon followed the lead of other regiments, giving up the French infantry red trousers they had at first adopted and turning to khaki or grey, and steel helmets.

Throughout the course of the war exotic, defining features of uniform dress were gradually eroded.

***

Looking at some of the vagaries of uniform worn by both Central Powers and Allied troops, it is remarkable how similar the basic new field grey and khaki uniforms were, in terms of both design and finish. This may be due in part to the influence of German tailoring in London,[89] combined with the growing importance of Paris as a centre of design. Moreover, while traditional clothing and existing fashion had some influence on military uniforms, conversely uniform had a marked effect on civilian styles. Clothes that had proved practical in the trenches were not only translated into non-military designs because they were more comfortable or durable, but also because they were found aesthetically appealing. Indeed, they often became less practical in translation. The curious mix of a noble chivalric past and present bloody danger, evoked, for some, an unbeatable *élan*.

3 MEN IN CIVVIES;
WOMEN IN UNIFORM

If a man were of fighting age, but for whatever reason not in uniform, then decisions about dress could be difficult. To be out and about in a civilian suit was met with suspicion, and sometimes outright animosity. Women in jobs never before available to them, had also to find a new way of dressing. Where the war effort required, the uniforms women wore in factories, trades and as nurses and ancillary staff, were a manner of rebuke to those non-uniformed men. The genders were set against each other through the medium of dress.

Some men remained civilian yet dressed themselves in the manner of soldiers. The war artist François Flameng, living it up at Maxim's restaurant in Paris, responded to 'the gravitational pull of the military world'[1] with his own quasi-uniform, 'wearing a kepi, a khaki jacket with rows of medal ribbons on the chest and puttees'.

The impact of uniform on male dress was more often insidious, for fashion can creep up on us, even if we imagine ourselves immune. The belted Norfolk jacket, for example, had been popular sporting wear in the Edwardian era, and fashionable among the up-and-coming middle classes who wanted to ape the appearance of the sporting gentleman, whether or not they actually went hunting, shooting and fishing themselves. In this period the jacket rather than the frockcoat became more everyday. It mimicked military versions with its many buttoned pockets, particularly when worn with plus fours tucked into boots, again suggesting not so much a man of business, or for that matter of leisure, but a man of action.

Aspects of military garb are present in post-war men's fashion, such as the Burberry mackintosh (mentioned in Chapter 2), but even during the course of the war the desire for a greater definition of shoulder, the suggestion of a figure trimmed lean through manly exertion, hair worn shorter than before the war with whiskers less abundant, suggesting less vanity and more practicality. It might have seemed implicitly unpatriotic to dress otherwise and the layman might well have hoped to enjoy some of the respect attached to military uniform thereby.

It was important, were he not to seem merely foolish or self-deluded, to suggest rather than to seem dressed up in military fancy dress, wearing elements of former wars say, to demonstrate that a man had paid his dues in the past. This might on occasion have been a ploy to avoid the critical eye of those who sought to shame the coward, but more often such men, particularly those invalided out or too old or somehow deemed unsuitable to serve, were inclined to seek the comfort of understated but military style clothing.

At the same time, a certain degree of resistance to military-styles grew up, in reaction to these quasi-uniform motifs. The informal lounge suit, already popular pre-war, took hold in America, Australia and New Zealand, and among younger men in Europe. It was a style that seemed to put comfort first, with the body of the man beneath hidden by its looser cut. Moreover, the new ready-to-wear market found the simple shape easier to mass-produce, since they did not need to fit closely. New soft collared shirts did not require the same degree of upkeep as starched wing collars. There were serious fabric shortages due to the priority given to uniform manufacture. Suit jackets tended to be cut a little shorter during the war years, sleeves and trouser legs narrower and elaborations on non-military jackets, such as belts, pleats and patch pockets gradually fell out of favour.[2] That said, what motivated someone to choose either a more uniform style or a loose cut unadorned suit is more likely due to a desire to appear either in on the action or modestly less extravagant in the context of a world at war.

For some men the war posed a profoundly difficult question. Conscientious objectors might agree to non-combatant service at home or abroad, wearing uniform in ancillary labour roles or, say, joining the Quakers' Friends' Ambulance Unit in the field. However, when men unwilling to fight but prepared to submit to conscription were brought into the war, many conscientious objectors feared that they were effectively forcing others into battle, having taken up the non-combatant roles themselves. The alternative was prison, where conditions were severe. Some objectors refused prison work that might in any way support the war effort, so that for example they might agree to sew mailbags, but not coal sacks that were intended for the Royal Navy. At such a time it must have been near impossible to avoid jobs that did not in some way support the war, for presumably mailbags were used to carry mail to the front, for instance, thus keeping up fighting morale.

British military authorities, frustrated by their refusal to conform, shipped a token 50 objectors to France, so that they would then be subject to military discipline. The ringleaders were given severe field punishments, such as a form of crucifixion – Field Punishment Number 1 – where they were tied to a beam or barbed wire for long periods, to break the spirit. Finally the men were lined up and sentence of death was pronounced. Only at the last minute was this commuted to penal servitude for ten years, after the British Prime Minister Asquith interceded on their behalf,[3] a case where a refusal to wear uniform had almost brought about execution.

There were those who were alive to the injustice of organizations such as the Active Service League, set up by Mrs Montague Barstow,[4] and the greater part of Mrs Pankhurst's Suffragette Movement, both of which barracked non-uniformed men of apparent fighting fitness for cowardice. Christabel Pankhurst called for military conscription for men and toured America in October 1914, encouraging the government there to join the war; Mrs Pankhurst herself visited Russia in an attempt 'to keep their wavering menfolk in the war'.[5]

There were British men occupied in essential civilian work or for health reasons unable to fight, who had to face women bent on shaming them. Some men targeted were already part of the military but on leave and wearing civilian clothes. In 1915 a man briefly back from the trenches has to leave off his uniform because it is lice-ridden. He goes out to a music hall and recalls:

As I lined up outside a lady came along and put a white feather into my hand … I felt small enough … but as I went into the gallery a chap came out in naval uniform … and said that no girl should be sitting with a chap unless he was in uniform.[6]

Another, a British sailor, home on leave after being torpedoed and just managing to survive, is also 'feathered', but claims he 'just took it in his stride'.[7]

The poet Helen Hamilton derides those who set out to humiliate men, without necessarily knowing the reason for those 'Who look in their civilian garb/Quite stout and hearty.'[8] She does not, however, defend men who are pacifist. The idea, reinforced by propaganda at the time, that women's role was to encourage men to war, must have led all too easily to a sense of righteous anger against those who appeared to shirk their duty as men. These men further offended by resisting female appeal.

The white feather was a long-established symbol of cowardice in Britain, stemming from the adage that a fighting bird with white feathers in its tail was of inferior stock, and thus unfit to fight. Reversing this idea, a white feather came to be used as a pacifist emblem, and later in the 1960s was adopted as a symbol of courage by American troops in Vietnam, when to wear a white feather in your hat was intended as a taunt to enemy snipers. Even during the First World War it had alternative meanings. The notion of panache, or stylish swagger, is – like Cyrano de Bergerac's gallantry – derived from a flamboyant white feather, like those worn in the cocked hats of Italian officers of the *Alpini* (discussed in Chapter 2).

Women and Military Style

While women not in uniform did not invite censure, military motifs on women's clothing became fashionable as the war progressed. There had been a vogue for oriental details, such as tassels and jewel colours in the wake of the Crimea, before the blazing influence of the Russian ballet. The First World War's effect was more pervasive, and khaki became for a while the new black for women's suits with trench-coat type coats with military adjustable button collars. In contrast, evening wear fought to maintain a sense of delicacy, this disparity confirming what Roland Barthes terms the essential fashion oppositions of 'weight and lightness, openness and closure, emphasis and neutrality'.[9]

One Scottish aid worker remarks on the sudden change in women's appearance,

> dressed in military, half-military or quarter-military dress, imaginative imitations of uniforms, perhaps a big, ill-fitting greatcoat, 'thrown open with a large belt at the back'.[10]

When women did adopt uniform their motives could be in doubt. In one *Punch* cartoon of 1916, for example, a woman excitedly tries on her new uniform, primping and preening in front of a full-length mirror. Her husband looks on amused, confident that nothing has changed after all, and that women are still as silly as ever about their appearance.

Women working at the front, even when in para-military dress, tended to be given soft caps to wear, though there are many photographs of nurses wearing steel helmets. Though I have not seen this anywhere specifically mentioned, it is likely that discarded helmets were picked up along the way and worn for safety, and even style. Russian and Serbian female soldiers on the other hand were issued with helmets, marking out their higher status as warriors.

Some women, far from aping the image of men in action, preferred what they wore to look different from the new uniforms, with their less tailored silhouette. They opted to retain what they felt to be their allure – their difference from men – and thus look in contrast, less capable of practical activity. This look was therefore more restrictive, such being the contrary nature of fashion:

When men were slope-shouldered, like First World War soldiers, women adopted padded shoulders to enhance the trim feminine waist.[11]

For women, hoping to gain ground in secretarial and administrative jobs, it was important to seem, and therefore to appear, competent. Clerical work had been a rare category of respectable, non-manual, non-domestic work for women prior to the war, but wages were low even though they were 'expected to manage to dress themselves like ladies'.[12] A sack-shaped suit would not do, or rather it needed to be adapted to the female form. The look was business-like in its sober coloured, un-flimsy suiting with more feminine blouses in artificial silks and fine cotton.

In London, department stores had to contend with customers concerned it might appear unpatriotic if they were seen to be concerned with new clothes at such a time. As well as avoiding the display of garments that seemed inappropriately ornate, 'in all the tasteful window displays there was hardly a frill or a furbelow to be seen', Harrods demonstrated its sensitivity with:

> demonstrations of bandage-making and a cutting-out service for flannel bed jackets suitable for wounded soldiers and expert staff would be on hand to give advice on the selection of knitting wool and patterns for garments for the troops.[13]

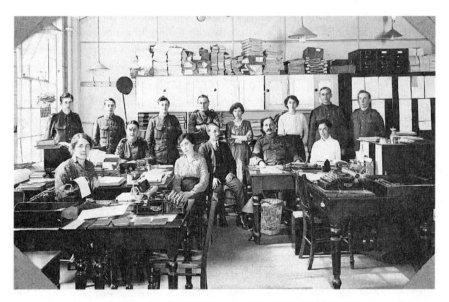

13. Office staff of King George V Military Hospital, Stamford Street, London, c.1915.

Yet far from being a period when women of means were inclined to avoid new clothes, the new crinoline shaped skirts became all the rage across Europe. In Germany the *Kriegskrinoline*, a term for the suit silhouette that dominated from 1915 to 1917, had its skirts at first supported by layers of frothy petticoat. Other versions of this full shape are the multi-layered pannier skirt, and as fashion tends to the extreme, culminating in the barrel skirt of 1917, wide at the hip but narrow enough at the ankle to restrict easy movement, as with the hobble skirt prior to the First World War.

In uniforms designed for active service, simply narrowing and shortening the full shaped skirt allowed major savings in yardage once fabric shortages began to bite.

The difficulty in getting supplies within Germany, caused by the Allied shipping blockade, meant that ingenuity was required if you wanted a new dress or pair of shoes. As the war progressed everything that could be recycled was, cutting down adult clothes for children and using any fabric source available. Piete Kuhr, the young girl from Schneidemühl, dreams of having two beautiful outfits for her confirmation, but what is possible fails to delight. For her examination she is given a piece of ersatz silk, which 'looks just like those silky-shining, glistening sticky sweets with stripes right through ... bonbon red with white and green', that she is forced to wear with an old black skirt of her aunt's. And for the confirmation itself:

> Grandmother had sacrificed a brown and green curtain ... decorated with a narrow black braid ... a half-length dress with a waist, long sleeves and a little round cut-out at the neck ... I looked at her and thought that I loved her above all, and that it was disgraceful of me to cry with disappointment.[14]

Any leather available was required for military purposes, so Piete and her friends have to make do with cloth sandals with soles made of wood, in three sections for flexibility, and held together with strips of recycled leather. One disadvantage was that they made a clattering noise, and Piete dreams of daintier footwear. With the slightly shorter skirts, button boots left an unsightly portion of leg between boot and skirt hem, so increasingly shoes with a small heel were preferred. On the day of Piete's confirmation she is delighted to be presented with a charming pair of fabric shoes. As she joins her classmates in the old black skirt and artificial silk blouse, yet feeling rather grand with 'Grandmother's black 1862 hymn book with gilt edging; a delicate lace handkerchief had come from Aunt Emma Haber in Berlin, and Grandmother had made a little cross out of real violets and placed it on the handkerchief' and wearing the pretty, lightweight shoes, she is astonished when children laugh and point at her in the street, shouting out 'Coffin shoes!' Her grandmother had bought them from the local undertaker. They are shoes for corpses in their coffins.

The French POW Gaston Riou remarks disparagingly on the villagers' clothes at his prison in Bavaria, when they come to gawp at him and his fellow prisoners, clearly lacking, in his opinion, a certain *je ne sais quoi*:

> In their Sunday best, wearing cocks' feathers in their green felt hats; rich farmers' wives trying to look comfortable in hats; swarms of children for the most part barefooted; peasants in ill-fitting ready-made clothes; pathetic village dames, clad as in Dürer's pictures, the head covered with a kerchief, a black fichu over the shoulders, a wadded corsage to fill out their figures. All these idlers looking poverty stricken when compared with those of like class in France, would spend hours staring at the 'pantalons rouges'.[15]

Those women of the lower middle class, in both Britain and Germany, who took up clerical jobs, faced a society that was accustomed to esteem women on the basis of their physical attractions, however much they might prefer to be valued for their business proficiency. Cheryl Buckley, looking at women's role in the war through the glass of the inexpensive magazine *Home Chat*, finds that 'fashion functioned as *the* key representational site where women from the skilled working class and lower middle class in Britain began to make visible their changing consciousness and identities'.[16] She reveals the magazine's attempts to both stand aloof from fashion at such a time, and then quickly and without embarrassment embrace it again:

> Nobody is thinking about fashion just now, but most of us will soon be thinking about a pretty blouse ... a women's duty is to try and make herself as nice as she can.[17]

This may seem a contradiction, but its rub – the dilemma of wanting to be taken seriously but also seem appealing – still holds true for women today. Some working-class women might have escaped domestic servitude to enjoy better wages and a measure of social freedom working on buses, in munitions factories and in telecommunication related jobs for example, but they still wanted to be found attractive. The uniforms of domestic staff had often been appreciated by girls previously more poorly clad, particularly if entering a reasonably prosperous household and enjoying a new dress for the first time. Those working below stairs would have had a simple cotton dress provided, plain coloured or often striped, with a plain apron, collar, sleeve-tidies and cap. If they were used for upstairs duties also (as a between-stairs, or 'tweeney') there would be a change to a frillier apron and cap. Housemaids and ladies' maids fared rather better in their flattering black dresses as described rather wistfully by a kitchen maid many years later:

> The maids were very smart. They had tight sleeves … puffed … built up … tight jackets, little buttons right down the front to a peak … and long skirts. They looked ever so smart. Nice caps.[18]

The new women's uniforms could be far from alluring. One West London bus conductor describes the discomfort and nuisance of her heavy suit:

> a very thick sergey material, in a very dark navy blue, with a skirt coming off, I suppose, from about 12–15 inches from the ground, and a tunic coat … [like] the old Norfolk jackets, with two rows of things over the shoulder [and] a belt come through … and buttons down the front … and two leather straps across the shoulders … a kind of hat with a strap under the shoulder, and gaiters … that strapped underneath our insteps … and they came nearly up to the knee … you can imagine that on your early turn in the morning, strapping up those things … lacing them up like lace boots, but going twice as far, they were a blinking nuisance really! But it was your uniform … in the winter we had overcoats to put over our uniform … They were really cumbersome.[19]

An important distinction (mentioned in Chapter 2) is the lack of colour in male dress, and in this respect women's uniform was masculine. In Western culture, the variety and colourfulness of female dress, for women of sufficient means to afford impractical and often expensive colour in delicate silk, chiffon and lace, had been in contrast to male black or sombre clothing. Now the war was to encourage women into grave, dark uniform, even if they might privately long for some delightful divergence from complete uniformity. Others, who wanted to be taken seriously in the workplace but did not have a prescribed uniform, chose to create their own versions of masculine tailored suits.

Military influences that were taken up by women include features such as silk cravats, echoing an earlier age of male splendour, along with, say, scarlet and vermillion piping on dark coloured travelling suits, sailor suits mimicking naval uniform and a wide variety of army and naval hat styles. Costume jewellery was often reminiscent of honorary medals, not to mention the trend for both trench art jewellery pieces and those made to look as if they had been fashioned from wire and shell casings. German women were encouraged to give up their gold wedding rings for the war effort, and were given in return replacements made of iron, inscribed with the word

Vaterlandsdank (Fatherland thanks),[20] a case of less sumptuous jewellery bearing a higher status.

One journalist at the time commented that the war had achieved a new military bearing in women:

> One of the uses of this appalling war will be, that we have had the rarest of opportunities for the expressing of beautiful *ligne*.[21]

Where women adopted uniforms, it suggested a new independence, disallowing men's vicarious pleasure in the sumptuous costume of their dependent womenfolk. However, wearing uniform can also suggest a subservient position to both wearer and observer, which may in turn explain why women, with their history of lower status, were sometimes eager to subvert in small ways the uniforms they had struggled to gain. VAD uniforms were uncomfortable, with tight starched collars, belts and 'awful studs that went flying all over the place',[22] though these standards were often dropped in the field. Their dresses were meant to be worn long, to the ankle, but ignoring the admonishing eye of matron, young women with an eye for fashion turned up their hems as high as they dared.[23]

Despite the divide between officer and lower ranks, which fed into the hierarchies of new female jobs and organizations at home and abroad, it is sometimes claimed that the war brought aristocracy and clerks, shop assistants and domestic servants into closer proximity. However, though for men of fighting age the challenge of the war theatre was almost inevitable, many women remained in domestic service, their lives undergoing very little change at all – for it was only a minority who took up war work. Women's desire to contribute their labour[24] may have been sincere, but there were, certainly at the beginning of the war, relatively few opportunities. In Britain, orphanages such as Snaresbrook Asylum in East London, had long had the custom of dressing their boys in military style uniforms and marshalling them in cadet-style corps, so that they were easily recruited into the forces at 16, whereas girls were dressed in the manner of domestic servants and trained in cooking, cleaning and needlework, in preparation for a life in service.

In Germany, the desire to participate in frontline work also far outweighed available jobs.[25] Many lower middle-class women remained in their traditional roles, caring for their families or working in shops, in dressmaking and small scale manufacturing jobs, just as they had done before the war. On the Continent a greater proportion of women lived in rural communities and day-to-day life remained very much as it had always been. In Germany and France, Bulgaria and Serbia, women living in the countryside, with their men gone off to war, were drawn into greater co-operation with women on neighbouring farmsteads, so that in this sense the war brought about a social revolution in their lives. There may have been limited funds and insufficient outside influence to allow any obvious change in dress, but interaction, and the effect of soldiers and ancillary staff passing through their villages, did begin to undermine many long held attitudes regarding what was appropriate wear. Thick dark peasant skirts, dragged down in winter with the mud of hard labour; stifling corsets and close bonnets at harvest: to an idle bystander they might have looked much the same in 1918 as before the war, yet a skirt an inch or two shorter and an easing up of old modesties must have felt like a significant change to those women.

The majority of women from all classes who were able to enjoy new job opportunities, nonetheless, remained in the class in which they had entered the war, even if greater financial independence allowed new clothes' buying, making them appear more similar, at a cursory glance at least. Newspaper advertisements for domestic staff, for instance, on both sides of the conflict, display a preference for reasonably young but experienced staff. No doubt this has always been true, yet these were the very women with sufficient confidence to risk turning their backs on old ways, daring to take up new, better paid work opportunities.

For the upper-class woman bent on supporting her country, the war offered an opportunity and release from the boredom of a life without purpose, beyond finding a suitable husband or producing an heir. It might mean the business of forming committees and fund-raising. If they were drawn into more direct contact with soldiers at home or abroad, then there was the question of how to dress while tending to the needs of the wounded or raising the spirits of convalescents – providing new fashion opportunities.

Lynette Powell, of Queen Alexandra's Imperial Military Nursing Service (QAIMNS) was posted to a hospital in le Touquet, where the presiding Duchess cut a splendid figure on the wards, with her wolfhound in attendance. Powell describes the Duchess and her friends as keen to meet the convoys of wounded men when they first arrived:

'It's the least we can do to cheer up the men' the Duchess always used to say … even if it were 9.00 in the morning [they] went upstairs and changed into full evening dress, with diamond tiaras and everything … They meant very well but it did look funny, these ladies all dressed up and the men, all muddy on the stretchers, looking at them as if they couldn't believe their eyes.[26]

There are accounts of well-to-do women in Paris throwing themselves into nursing, while remaining at the cutting edge of fashion, Madame Henri de

Rothschild accessorizing her uniform with a beautiful pearl collar. Mrs 'Willie K' Vanderbilt had white piqué uniforms tailored at the House of Worth, adding a gold and ruby cross, hung on a tassel, for a touch of added bling.[27] These women were spending long hours nursing seriously wounded men, but they still wanted to enjoy dress and accessory.

In a semi-biographical account of ambulance drivers in the field, uniform regulations lose out to the tawdry necessities of women living in difficult conditions at close quarters. Tosh, the niece of an earl, appears to support the idea of the British aristocracy being somehow above fashion concerns – as was sometimes the case in munitions factories, as we shall see. She wanders 'in the flickering candlelight in a soiled woollen undervest and a voluminous pair of navy blue bloomers'. Another woman is distressed that, as she dies, her treasured Burberry mackintosh is getting stained with blood. She[28] feels that her fetching uniform has been utterly wasted:

> in a place where the men are too wounded or too harassed to regard women other than cogs in the great machinery, and the women are too worn out to care whether they do or not.[29]

Sister Joan Martin-Nicholson, in Warsaw in 1914, reviled nurses from Poland and Russia for wearing 'tweed, cotton or silk shirts topped with lace, cotton or satin blouses ... according to the wearer's station in life'.[30] She felt that a nurse's status required the strict formality of uniform.

Women in Uniform

Those women who took on physical labour such as heavy duty work in coalmines, in factories such as the Pimlico depot in London where the vast majority of army clothing was made from 'boots and socks up to ceremonial scarlet uniforms',[31] or in rough trades such as wheel tapping, plumbing, electrical work, telephone instillation and brewing say, all needed suitable clothing to meet the new conditions. In civilian women's dress, the soft belted over-tunic that had accompanied the pre-war fashion for narrow skirted suits, was adapted for more practical purposes by the simple expedient of removing the under-skirt and lengthening the over-skirt to form a pleated skirt which allowed for easy movement.[32] The silhouette echoes that of a lower-ranks' male uniform, and can be seen mirrored in the cut of female postal workers, police officer's navy, First Aid Nursing Yeomanry (FANY) and VAD ambulance drivers, Women's Legion drivers and the Women's Army Auxiliary Corps (WAAC) in their khaki gabardine.

Although women, working in what had been male domains, were a challenge to conventional notions of appropriate feminine behaviour, the need for their labour meant that they were at least publicly encouraged in Britain. In Germany, however, despite a similar need, there was initially a lack of official advertising for female auxiliary staff, the War Office fearing too great a disruption to the labour market. As it was mainly working-class women who were drawn into clerical and domestic war work, in mess kitchens say, the fact that they were not uniformed, to save cloth it was said, resulted in 'far-reaching consequences for their public perception, as there were practically no identifiable images of them in the press'.[33]

Without uniform's badge of respect, female auxiliary workers in Germany were easy to vilify as spendthrifts, improved wage packets said to be feeding 'an addiction to new clothes', economic freedom allowing greater social freedom which in turn led to accusations of moral decline. While a Colonel Bauer expressed his distaste for the 'extended self-adulation [and] ridiculous gushing' over women's war work, Agnes von Harnack, who organized auxiliary recruitment from late 1917, has yet sterner concerns:

> In former times an army was openly accompanied by prostitutes. With our modern ideas of what a woman should be, of her dignity and worth, we could not overlook the danger entailed in sending out girls of different social background to supply the army.[34]

For 'different social background' here it is not clear whether she is referring solely to working-class women, or to the possibility of middle-class women becoming contaminated. Not all auxiliary workers were uneducated, and women of the higher social standing bourgeoisie, the *Bildungsbürgertum*, were, for example, employed as translators, and widely approved of as 'fine, elegantly dressed ladies'.

The British Queen Mary is pictured visiting munitions factories and awarding medals to women who had been injured or honouring those killed. The workers' clothing lacked the marginally smarter delineation of military uniform, yet its smocks[35] and trousers, and even puttees, created a common identity amongst the women. However, an ambulance driver in East Africa wrote home to his fiancée in England, warning her against wearing trousers, implying that such clothing would diminish his desire for her:

> I hope you don't wear trousers on your job, sweetheart – I think it's so disgusting.[36]

Such an obviously gender-transgressing garment as trousers was 'so widely represented in the press that it became a recognized cultural icon'.[37] French

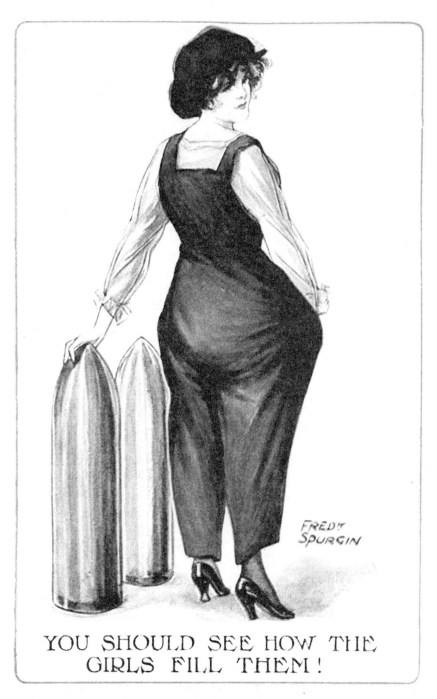

YOU SHOULD SEE HOW THE
GIRLS FILL THEM!

14. Women in trousers could amuse and even arouse distaste. Fred Spurgin postcard of a munitions worker in dungarees and mobcap, worn with high heels and pretty blouse.

women visiting provincial munitions factories in Britain were so impressed with 'your women's neat and common-sense trousers and plain, workmanlike coats'[38] that they took samples home to copy.

Munitions workers' hair and skin could become stained a virulent yellow if exposed to TNT (trinitrotoluene, an explosive agent), which led to their nickname of 'canaries'. In fact the long-term effects of such powerful chemicals could be serious, toxic jaundice being evidence of possible blood and organ tissue damage.[39] A woman observing workers at the time recalls their strange appearance as unfeminine. Note the reference below to the Amazons, the mythical women who significantly allowed their bodies to be exposed in defiance of male supremacy:

> Amazonian beings ... bereft of all charm of appearance, clothed anyhow, skin stained a yellow-brown even to the roots of their dishevelled hair ... Were these really women?[40]

Yet the unnaturally lurid colouring was something many of these women wore with pride, a mark of their dangerous role, and reminiscent of the superstition some men felt against wiping their faces clean of mud and blood in the heat of battle. Sometimes the yellow dye was found unflattering, even by a more sympathetic audience:

> My older sister, she went to the Arsenal ... She was all yellow and to crown it all she was ginger ... so what with her ginger hair and yellow skin![41]

Alice Connor recalled other dangers, in the production of fuses and the rather inadequate means of protection available:

> We had caps to cover our hair, and to stop the hot brass hitting our necks we turned our collars up.[42]

A desire for decoration was not allowed to extend to jewellery, including wedding rings or metal buttons, since they could spark off an explosion. Even hairgrips were prohibited, and forgetfulness was no defence, so that whether an oversight or not, any infringement faced the shame of a 28-day prison sentence and summary dismissal.

However, a variety of small nuances of dress came to signify different work teams or roles within a workforce, such as carefully arranging the angle of the protective mobcaps worn or pinning posies to smocks, with each 'shop' having its own flower emblem or design of stocking.[43] One popular trend was for wearing brightly coloured ribbons instead of government-issued shoelaces:

First the 'cap shop' girls strutted proudly with emerald green ribbons in their shoes, the 'new fuse' girls followed with yellow, and soon the whole Arsenal was in the fashion.[44]

Arnold Bennett, visiting one of the factories, rhapsodized about women workers in trousers 'with an elaborate white lacy corsage or a flowing, glowing scarf', one girl who 'rolled a nine inch shell over her fashionable glacé kid boot that peeped out beneath the yellow overall' somehow managing to catch his eye.[45] Despite their rough work, these women and their attention to the detail of dress clearly struck Bennett as romantic, even beguiling, their new economic freedom giving them the opportunity to indulge in the fripperies of fashion:

I spends the whole racket
On good times and clothes.
… Years back I wore tatters,
Now – silk stockings, mi friend![46]

Although uniform smocks were required in the munitions factories, when it came to what was worn outside working hours, there were wages to be spent and a wide range of dress styles. Some who considered themselves a cut above resented the factory workers' affluence, expressed through dress:

They had uniforms and mobcaps … and were given such money that, when they came out for their free time, they bought fur coats, all kinds of trinkets and gauzy scarves. It probably wasn't real fur – some of it was musquash – they flaunted themselves in the tubes [the underground trains in London].[47]

It was not only working-class women who had taken to working in these factories:

Some prefer tweeds remarkable for their absence below the knee, shooting boots and leather gaiters, but many incline to satin and *crêpe de Chine* of vivid hues, white kid boots, ostrich plumes, and no gloves … The few really shabby ones are popularly supposed to be peeresses.[48]

With money for clothes in the hands of working women who previously had had very much less surplus income, and more affluent classes happy to appear dowdy at times, previous class distinctions in terms of appearance became confused. Whereas the working-class women might now have the means to dress up, the upper and upper middle-class women could enjoy 'dressing up to their "normal" social position and dressing down to demonstrate their patriotism and commitment to the war effort'.[49] In effect a rare case of downward fashion mobility until our own top-down times, when it has become fashionable to mix high-end clothes with Primark throwaway additions.

For those women not in uniform it became fashionable to dress practically, avoiding apparently new clothes. Cheryl Buckley argues that a new 'chic stylishness' was both 'unstructured [and] slightly unruly' and that readers of the magazine *Home Chat* located their new independence in this new way of dressing.[50] However, she contends that those women who forgot their obligation to attract, and dressed accordingly, were damned for a lack of coquetry:

> Immodesty might sometimes be amusing, but the suggestion of sexual indifference was always intolerable.[51]

Some authorities were slow to allow women's uniforms to be designed with female body-shape in mind, and the resulting resentment was matched by the ingenuity some spent in adjusting the fit of overalls and baggy jodhpurs, say. The first uniforms issued for the Women's Royal Naval Service (WRNS), for example, were an ankle-length wrap-around dressing gown style in thick, scratchy navy serge, with miniature sailor collars that were cut uncomfortably high to the throat. Women would turn their collars back or beg and borrow male collars. To top the outfit off, they had pudding-basin style hats with a pleated crown. Officers at least fared a little better, with a more tailored cut and a more fetching tricorn black hat.[52]

Some women took to trousers, and many were shocked to see female farm workers happily wearing their breeches off duty. It can be tempting to map each alteration in dress to a conscious change in attitude, but change is more insidious. Conservative taste seemed to dictate that it was better to expose legs to view, rather than keep them covered but admit they went all the way up to the top. The fuss that had been made about 'extravagantly short'[53] skirts, which were still at most six to ten inches off the ground, was nothing compared with the shock of seeing the length of women's legs, albeit clothed. Certainly older generations found the sight of women in masculine clothing troubling. A young cook asks a much older woman for a reference to join the Women's Land Army, and she exclaims:

> 'It means that you'll be dressed as a man! And I object to that ... It's a disgrace to show your ankles.' Of course it was, and I had very long skirts in those days.[54]

When the cook begins work on a farm outside Chichester, wearing her breeches and smock, another woman peers at her and remarks, 'Hmphh ...

Neither man nor woman!' At first the WLA recruits were reluctant to wear trousers:

> They made us sore. It was rough inside. They wasn't proper seams. They were raw inside. Of course you wore your underclothes, but it did [rub], in different places, under your knees, till you got used to it.[55]

These are practical rather than concerns to do with feminine shame. The WLA clothing could be uncomfortable in other ways, with no waterproof rubber boots provided, only hobnail boots, or for wet conditions clogs with wooden soles and leather uppers that took in rain through the eyelets. As no gloves were provided, the recruit wears old male socks to protect her hands when ploughing. Although Land Army workers received a new uniform every year from the government, which included a cap and mackintosh, and even though they were allowed very little free time, she still feels the need to buy herself a few smarter items for going to church. 'I bought a pair of brown brogue shoes ... my dress kit ... I got a pair of cotton gloves ... my walking-out,' evidence of a desire to look her best in uniform. She is happy to work hard and to wear what she is given, yet in the long hot summer of 1916 she is sweltering and comes to a decision:

> I was out in the field and wet through with sweat, and of course in those days there was corsets and all steel bones. All got rusty ... I took 'em off ... I throwed them down the outside lavatory they emptied every third year ... and from that day to this, never wore anything at all![56]

Before the war, women employed in coal mining, for instance, had worn trousers for work, but were never seen in them outside the pit gates. Over their trousers they would wear skirts, which were rolled up for work, and then let down for the journey home. There were attempts made by the British Country Women's Field Labour Committee to enforce 'ordinary feminine dress'[57] when the WLA were not working, but this was overruled by the governmental Country Agricultural Committee.

Aural records at Somerset County Library show that 'uniform' trousers were sometimes just what could be begged from husbands and fathers, and not regulation issue at all. However, the freedom trousers gave was not easily surrendered, even if it would be decades before women could wear trousers without inviting disapproval.

In Ireland, despite the split in support for the First World War caused by the delay in ratification of the Home Rule Bill, female uniforms for nationalist organizations like the *Cumann na mBan* bear a close resemblance to British uniforms, though they were of a darker khaki.[58] Countess Markievicz, who was involved in the Easter Rising of 1916, helped design uniforms for the Irish Citizen Army. She attended trial in uniform, and it was reported that, 'a lot of hatred ... seemed to be directed at the Countess's breeches'.[59]

***

Comparing the various details of clothing requirements of different service organizations, the ordered lists bring to life the women who must once have read them over and again, representing their new unknown life ahead, of how many pairs of socks and vests and handkerchiefs were prescribed, lending a dignity to toothbrush, comb and small mirror. Then years later these uniforms, or parts of uniform, are collected by museums whose curators make new lists. It is as if all that is left of an individual woman's service career is this brief document and the few items of dress that remain:

> Coat: buff or light khaki drill, single-breasted, long jacket type, 3 pockets, belt, straps on wrists, bust size 40"+; labels: '3' and 'A W Gamage Ltd., Holborn/ E C' Light brown buttons
> Breeches: whipcord, khaki, lacing at knees; waist 33"
> Breeches: buff drill, laced at knees, waist 40"+
> Shirt: cream-coloured linen, with loose collar, not matching in colour etc. Shirt is rather worn.[60]

The WLA handbook reminds these women that whatever they are wearing, they must strive to maintain their femininity, even if they are 'dressed rather like a man':

> remember, just because you wear a smock and breeches you should take care to behave like a British girl who expects chivalry and respect from everyone she meets.[61]

In Britain, the Home Office appointed female police officers to deal with the wave of crime amongst women, particularly in relation to prostitution around military camps. Their uniforms were designed to look as much like male officers as possible, heavy and uncomfortable 'with a long skirt' and tunic, leather belt and hard, unyielding boots 'up to our knees', with hats 'like army helmets'.[62] Make-up was forbidden as was any but the most severely styled hairstyle:

Not an atom, not even a stray end, showing itself from beneath the close-fitting helmet.[63]

Clothing designed for Glaswegian female bus conductors was more flattering, and the women were praised in the press for their 'natty uniforms in Black Watch tartan'.[64] As the war drew on, on both sides of the conflict, women's role became recognized as essential to keep society's infrastructure intact. In Prussia, female conductors and guards working on the railways, wearing wide-legged trousers, suggested to some that women might be seeking political as well as dress freedom. They might choose to wear more feminine clothes off duty, but there was a suspicion that:

there is a profound political development in the official wear of the too-obviously divided nether garment.[65]

The Women's Voluntary Reserve (WVR) was recruited in Britain mainly from the upper and upper middle classes. They regulated against wearing jewellery and low-necked blouses with their uniforms, as to do so was said to show 'a lack of good taste'. Uniform was 'not merely a form of dress [but] something to be respected'.[66] Each member had to pay £2 and more for their khaki uniforms, a sum which would have been difficult to find for less privileged women. The Marchioness of Londonderry noticed this, and went on to set up the Women's Legion, which had a wider appeal in part because it provided recruits with their uniform. Although in both cases the work was largely administrative, often to do with fund-raising, the clothing, through its similarity to male service uniform, was intended to give the women a sense of authority and fellowship with the men at war.

Nursing Uniform

The first nurses' training scheme had taken place in Prussia in the 1830s, instituted by Theodor and Friedericke Fleider,[67] who realized the need to distinguish recruits from religious orders and untrained domestic staff that had previously been the only nursing resource. The nurses' elegant dark blue dresses, with white collars and bonnets that tied under the chin, were intended to imbue these single women with an unassailable air of respectability. Uniforms were to be unadorned, the starched white linen suggesting both physical and moral purity:

their uniform clothing came to symbolize caring, professional competence, and above all, unquestionable moral character.[68]

In Germany *Freiwillige Krankenpflege*, or voluntary nursing, carried on the conservative tradition. The nurse's role in the First World War was seen as spiritual and maternal 'to care, love and give, hence creating true happiness, inner peace and everlasting satisfaction'.[69] As male nurses were increasingly called up to be soldiers, there was a growing need for female aides on active duty behind the lines and in recuperation hospitals, and these volunteers soon came to outnumber trained nursing staff. They were more closely regimented than Allied nurses on the whole, and like the British WVR, were expected to buy their own uniform. Since wages were low, it was thus only those of some means who could afford to join up.

Even if women were concerned to appear competent, they had to be careful to seem unassertive. Thus the success of the Almeric Paget Military Massage Corps – who offered the first physiotherapy treatments, then known as Massage and Electrical Current Treatment – depended on a tactical decision not to seem too keen to get out into the field of battle, keenness being seen as a masculine preserve. The APMMC was set up in 1915 to work in military hospitals and convalescent camps, but did not see active service overseas until 1917.[70] Though they drilled in military fashion in simple navy blue wool uniforms, it was their apparent reticence, aided by the femininity of their all-white ward uniform, which eventually disposed the authorities to allow them to work behind the lines. The white dresses and veils of a nun's robe and wimple worn by helpers at the Revigny canteen were even more arresting, as subtly glamorous as their medieval inspiration.[71]

The Meaning of Uniform

In a fine example of sartorial restraint, the British nurse Edith Cavell refused to appear at her trial for espionage in her smart navy uniform, to 'deflect any additional attention away from the [nursing] school'. Despite the favourable impression it would have given to the court, she felt that wearing her nursing uniform in order to persuade the authorities that she deserved special treatment would be an improper use of the mystique of her calling.

Her fellow nurse and member of the French and Belgian resistance, Marie de Croy, thought her modesty 'a pity' as 'anything in the way of uniform always impressed the German mind'.[72] Cavell thought it ironic to be in court dressed again in the civilian white blouse, blue skirt and coat that she had worn on first coming to Brussels. However, she allows herself one moment

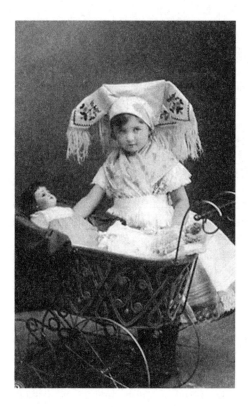

15. A little girl learning to nurture, in imitation uniform.

of pride, adjusting the two feathers on her hat before entering court, insisting that she 'might as well go out in style'.[73]

For many who volunteered, the mystique of the nursing uniform was what they sought. They yearned for the adventure and prestige of being behind the lines, imagining all manner of romance. One young VAD of 17 describes how she and her friends would bleach the red crosses on the front of their aprons in order to look as if they had been laundered many times, for she hoped to seem an old hand at saving lives. She and her fellow nurses would go to football matches in their spare time and 'sprinkle ourselves liberally with carbolic or ether, just so that there would be a hospital smell about us'.[74]

It was traditional for women to be seen as carers, and the chivalric air that was thought to surround the fighting man (as discussed in Chapter 2), was matched by the assumption of womanly grace in the nurse, an officer at the time voicing this connection:

I see them as great ladies, medieval in their saintliness, sharing the pollution of the battle with their champions.[75]

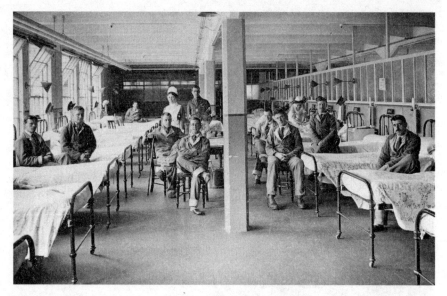

16. The King George Hospital for wounded soldiers, Stamford Street, London.

Nursing may have been a more acceptable role for women, but when they insisted on service in the field of battle, and in particular took to wearing khaki, then they provoked criticism. *The Ladies' Pictorial Magazine* of August 1915 decried women's ambition to wear masculine uniform:

> At this time when women are urging men to don this uniform, when they are rightly vaunting the glory and honour and distinction of wearing it, they themselves in many instances are rendering it ridiculous by adopting it themselves and playing at soldiers.[76]

British nurses, dressed for ward work in white aprons over pale cotton dresses, found that keeping clean in field hospital conditions was difficult. Their changes of dress were limited, and while aprons were relatively easy to wash themselves, the long sleeves with their separate over-sleeves or cuffs would quickly become saturated with blood and septic matter. With limited laundry facilities this was a constant problem. Danish nurses' uniforms, on the other hand, had short sleeves, allowing the forearm to be easily disinfected.[77]

It was a question of striking the right balance, between what was neither too suggestive nor too slovenly in appearance. In 1916, the British Journal of Nursing, *Pro Patria*, set out a standard that deftly undermines volunteer, untrained nursing staff:

To meet a Red Cross nurse in France wearing white silk stockings and high-heeled white shoes, shocks one's sense of propriety, just as to meet an English nurse with an untidy head, a waist faintly indicated by her apron strings, and ankles thickened by wrinkled stockings offends one's sense of patriotism.[78]

A VAD nurse, posted to the General Hospital in Rouen, is disgusted with the impracticality and ugliness of their uniform 'long black cloaks with little braid-edged shoulder capes; and small bonnets made of straw and trimmed with black velvet bows which were secured to our heads by narrow white strings'.[79] When America joined the Allies in April 1917, one nursing volunteer was so disappointed by the 'horrible looking uniforms of grey crèpe and aprons like butchers'[80] that she gets her mother to make her a smarter outfit, so much more flattering that other nurses would beg to borrow her aprons.

As the war drew on, women continued to adjust and sometimes completely transform their own uniforms. One British ambulance driver, for instance, claimed to have exchanged most of her uniform for more stylish French 'blue azure velvet breeches ... These plus a red *ceinture*',[81] (belt) insisting that this get-up had protected her from being shot, as her original khaki had been too much like the green-grey of Bavarian regiments, and thus had been a temptation to Allied snipers. However pointless such orders were, VADs were instructed that:

Uniforms were to be worn smartly and in a uniform way and not to suit the taste of the individual ... No additions or alterations, such as furs, veils, bowties, or shirt collars worn over the coat, are permissible.[82]

Conditions could be so bad that however regulated a uniform was intended to be, it was necessary to wear layer upon layer of clothing to keep warm enough to do one's work. At Rouen, Mrs Olive Dent describes what a nurse might need to wear for night duty:

Woollen garments piled on cocoon-like under her dress; a jersey over the dress and under the apron or overall, another jersey above the apron, a greatcoat, two pairs of stockings, service boots or gumboots with a pair of woolly socks, a sou'wester, mittens or gloves [perhaps both] and a scarf.[83]

Sometimes standard issue uniforms could be supplemented by locally available clothing. An English nurse working in Russia manages to buy a warm leather coat with a 'thick sheepskin waistcoat' for the coldest weather, known as a *dushegreychka* or soul-warmer, and since she will be riding in the

Carpathian mountains, she also gets hold of the dashing combination of black leather breeches and high boots.[84]

Less welcome than nurses at the front were female doctors such as Dr Elsie Inglis, of the Scottish Women's Hospitals, but when she and her colleagues made their own way into active service, the clothes they chose to adopt were again military in style. Dr Flora Murray and Dr Louisa Garrett, both militant suffragettes before the war and founders of the Women's Hospital Corps, wore full ankle length skirts and tunics in a greenish grey, and full-length overcoats. This quasi-uniform was topped off with small veiled hats, a nod to their superior standing as doctors, and to their femininity perhaps. Vera Brittain, alert to the details of dress, notes three elegantly suited 'lady doctors … in khaki tussore coats and skirts, dark blue ties and solar topees'.[85] There are also examples of doctors who insisted on maintaining their own individual ideas on style, such as one called Kitty, who 'appeared on her rounds … in frilly evening dresses reminiscent of a four-year-old at a party'.[86]

When America joined the conflict very few female doctors were allowed on active service either in the army or navy, and then only on the understanding that they remained officially civilian staff, even though they were in uniform. Thousands of American women volunteered for foreign service in 1917. Many served in non-military organizations such as the Salvation Army, both at home and in the field, and most wore uniform. For the dedicated officers of The Army, whose mission was to comfort men fighting in the bleak conditions of the trenches, living the same claustrophobic occasionally terrifying life, facing the discomforts of gas attack, intermittent sniper fire and even drowning in the sucking mud of Passchendaele say, clothes could seem important:

> They have not let these great things keep them from the pleasant little details
> of life. Even in the olive drab flannel shirt and serge skirt of their uniform, or in
> their trim serge coats, the exact counterpart of the soldier boy's, except for the
> scarlet epaulets, and the little close trench hat with its scarlet shield and silver
> lettering, they are beautiful and womanly. Catch them with the coat off and
> a great khaki apron enveloping the rest of their uniform, and you never saw
> lovelier women. No wonder they came to these girls with their troubles, or a
> button that needed sewing on.[87]

One Salvation Army officer found herself and her companions sleeping every night in a haystack, in order to be on the spot to support men transporting ammunition supplies under cover of darkness. The men noticed the increasingly shabby state of the women's uniforms, and took up a collection to buy them new garments. She objected, but finally agreed to take the money, not for new clothes, but to swell their fund for doughnuts and coffee for the men, instead.[88]

The National Society of Colonial Dames commemorated the work of female American volunteers by collecting the different uniforms worn, amounting to over a hundred, which are now housed in the collection of the National Museum of American History. They were struck by how important uniforms had been to the women, even to those playing a less dramatic role, such as librarians working in hospital libraries and dispatch offices. As with the nurses and doctors that came before them, they were 'equipped with uniform so that they may have standing with the military authorities and be given the respect and attention which an official connection with the military gives'.[89]

High status clothing has tended to be uncomfortable clothing, designed to demonstrate that the wearer has no need of easy, practical movement.[90] It might also be argued that clothing that demands immoderate attention, seeks high status. For instance, FANY drivers adopted distinctive tubular rabbit fur overcoats, lending them the appearance of 'mammoth hamsters'.[91] This was not only because they were extremely warm, but also the distinctiveness of their garments singled them out from other female participants in the war zone. The full cut goatskin fur coats were adopted despite being smelly when wet and attracting mud.[92] Similarly styled coats of 'extraordinary fullness' were worn in London, with military-type mitred caps and substantial leather gauntlets.

FANY uniform was otherwise rather haphazard. Earlier scarlet tunics and voluminous skirts cut for riding side-saddle gave way to a degree of informality, generally consisting of thick calf-length skirts and stout boots, augmented with 'silk scarves and snazzy gauntlets'.[93] Beryl Hutcheson describes her first uniform in 1915 of trousers and tunic with a skirt over the top fastened 'fore and aft' with press-studs,[94] the idea being that they were dressed ready to leap on a horse at a moment's notice, even though their designated work was to drive ambulances. FANYs were recruited from privileged classes and it seems likely that, as with upper-class women working in munitions, there remained a tendency to suggest their sense of confident superiority through such details of apparent sartorial negligence.

Female Soldiers

Some women had the gall to want to fight alongside men. While this was impossible in most armies, unless they pretended to be men,[95] in Russia women were actively recruited to form a force that might shame men grown weary of the war. The Battalion of Death, led by Maria Botchkareva, demanded a high standard of military discipline. They were given new standard issue male uniforms, of side-buttoned tunic and soft cap. One of their instructors reportedly compared them to Joan of Arc, who wore masculine dress into battle. Other Russian women's battalions were formed but never judged to be ready for combat, partly due to their lack of uniform provision. The First Women's Naval Detachment, for example, set up in 1917 by Maria Morskaia,[96] asked for boots and caps to be issued in smaller sizes, and even had tailors with sewing machines assigned to make the necessary alterations to their uniforms, but they were not popular with the authorities and were soon disbanded.

The Serbian army welcomed into its ranks a British woman, Flora Sandes, to fight alongside its men. She was permitted to dress as a man and subjected herself to the same rigorous life, often in freezing conditions in the mountainous regions of Macedonia. Compared with the nursing she had been doing, this new life gave her a greater sense of personal freedom and satisfaction. Yet just as the Bolsheviks ordered Russian women soldiers to return home and 'put on female attire' when they came to power, a wounded Sandes had little option but to return home to the restrictions of a woman's life, 'and a woman's clothes again'. Remarkably hardy during her wartime experience, years later she recalls her clothing with wry affection:

For evening dress, mud-stained, bloodstained khaki breeches and tunic, and for vanity bag a revolver.[97]

Peace at Last

When hostilities came to an end both men and women had to adapt to a world without war. A return to civilian clothing, and the continuing expectation for many women that they appear unfitted for strenuous labour, represented a troubling reversal. Men in the West, whether they had fought or not, could return to the sartorial safety of plain, dark, comfortable dress. Women still had to negotiate a way of dressing after uniform. For all its rigid regulations, its customizations and peculiarities, uniform had represented a period of extraordinary freedom for women.

4 THE FABRIC AND FURBELOWS

One day Mickey O'Shea stood in a trench somewhere
So brave, having a shave, and trying to part his hair.
'Take Me Back to Dear Old Blighty'[1]

There is a certain reluctance to think of the First World War in terms of grooming or attention to the details of dress. Yet, the pains people were prepared to go to for a stolen moment of luxurious indulgence, or perhaps just to retain some small aspect of home life, suggests that such pleasures were valued by the individual. An interest in the texture and colour of what was worn, its minor adjustments and embellishments, the longing for a cigarette, the confidence a new haircut gave or even something as minor as having sufficient hairpins to hand,[2] these matters affected people and helped them to endure. The experience of bathing skin that has been tormented by lice; a clean shave in comfortable circumstances after rationed water in a trench bunker; choosing a scent when the stench of the battlefield – of latrines with their overlay of chloride of lime, of septic wounds, or merely stale sweat in factory and field – these small pleasures could evoke a safer past and renew faith in a future state of peace.

For many, who before the war had enjoyed some privacy in their lives, even a few minutes taken to brush your teeth or to relieve yourself apart from others, 'the beauty of shitting in the open',[3] could seem important. Trench latrines, for example, were often communal, and consisted of a plank set over either a deep trench or just a bucket or biscuit tin, that then had to be emptied, often either as a punishment duty or by POWs.

When there was time to dig deep latrines away from living quarters, what was intended as a temporary resource could easily become more permanent, overflowing in wet weather and redolent of a 'never-to-be-forgotten' stench that for many represented trench life. Moreover, the longer a latrine was used the more risk was entailed:

Latrines were always dangerous places because of the regularity with which they had to be used [because of dysentery]. Jerry soon came to spot such places, and, believe me, they were not places to linger.[4]

Sometimes there was a lack of even these primitive arrangements:

We descended to primal man. No washing or shaving here, and the demands of nature answered as quickly as possible in the handiest and deepest shell-hole.[5]

Such acute sensory memory recalls the day-to-day business of war. The present moment experience of our dress is part of what it is to be human, intimately connected to the world of small impressions that sustain us. A nurse watching over severely wounded men at a clearing station one day, must have thought to offer a soldier her freshly laundered handkerchief, and thereafter this became her practice:

Whenever I have a very ill patient generally abdominal I always give him a clean handkerchief. I don't know why, but they love to have it.[6]

The folded, ironed linen must have seemed to represent to the men both maternal care and a future when such small features of civilization might be relevant again.

Production of fabric for the war effort had to come before the demands of personal preference or fashion. Shortages could have consequences in the field of battle, leading to the removal of identification numbers on German soldiers' helmet covers for example, when green cloth stocks ran low. Fine cotton netting produced for women's collars and light summer dresses pre-war, were made up into mosquito nets to relieve the irritation of flies and avoid the risk of infection to wounded men lying in makeshift hospital beds in Sevastopol.[7]

***

Luxury materials from Austro-Hungarian Galicia, German Silesia or from the British Derbyshire mills could still supply the wealthy in Paris, Berlin and London to more frivolous ends, but they were becoming more expensive and skilled dressmakers were increasingly difficult to find. Moreover, as the war developed, wearing fancy stuffs could in some circumstances become a sensitive issue (as discussed in Chapter 2). Cunnington suggests this accounts for an increasing lack of 'frills and furbelows'.[8] It is as if the continued presence of obviously luxurious fabric stands in fluttering contrast to the brutalities of the war. The poem 'Chemin des Dames' compares a battlefield with an elegant royal parade of the distant past, when the daughters of Louis XV, Adélaïde and Victoire, had regularly taken a path across what was now a battlefield. 'In silks and satins the ladies went',[9] as if the soldier poet had a sense of those princesses in their finery, as he fought for his life on the same ground 250 years later.

One young woman, stationed in Flanders, found learning the local art of lace-making an engrossing way of relieving the stress of frontline nursing:

> Some quite badly wounded people in. I learnt another stitch in lace-making a half stitch and made about six inches of lace in the night.[10]

It is touching to think that a cottage industry responsible for the fine lace headdresses of northern French peasant women, and that had once adorned the aristocrats of the court of Louis XIV, had all but died out by the beginning of the war. The eight lace-making schools in Bailleul had closed down due to the competition of new cheap machine-made lace, yet this nurse found herself drawn to that ancient craft.

In Paris, despite its proximity to the Western Front, fashionable life continued in extraordinary parallel. Where there was a shift from fancy silks and chiffons to cotton, linen and wool on account of availability, then the more practical look became fashionable. Yet, when Idina Sackville is in Paris shopping for haute couture in 1917, the *salons d'essayage*, or trying on rooms, were still able to complete a made to measure order in eight days, 'cut, stitched, embroidered, fitted and *fini*'. She finds Lanvin still 'overflowing with samples of silks, muslins and beadings in the latest designs, its eighty seamstresses' fingers still flying in its ateliers'.[11] James Laver discusses the upper-class set in Monte Carlo and the Mediterranean at the time waiting for the tiresome war to be over, with their taste for fine fabrics, for crêpe de chine, chiffon, mousseline and tulle in 'pastel shades or black with sequins'. They tried to avoid any change to their way of life, and the purchase and enjoyment of sumptuous clothing allowed them to hope that things might continue very much as they had before the war. However, even in this small sector of affluent society, the influence of wartime restrictions was felt, expressed in a preference for what was '*très simple, très chic*'.

Fabric does not necessarily provide comfort or pleasure. Its texture, or its deficiency to protect or suit weather conditions, can be singularly distressing. In the novel *Birdsong*,[12] a response to the invasive stench of rotting fabric in the trenches stands for a soldier's emotional and moral response to his situation. The protagonist, Stephen Wraysford, had worked in the cloth industry before the war, so that when he falls for a young woman, his attention is drawn to the fabric of her clothing as much as to the flesh beneath. The fabric itself comes to represent a longed for sensual delight beyond the war.

The Raw Materials

Walter Rathenau, head of the electronics firm AEG from 1915, was put in charge of German raw materials and had to contend with both the British naval blockade impeding supplies from the East and America, and also with difficulties transporting linen from Russia, which had suffered from a failed flax harvest in 1916.[13] High-quality linen was essential for aircraft bodies, for it needed to be strong enough to withstand the 'dope' coating of cellulose acetate to make them waterproof and wind resistant.[14] The Central Powers occupied many of the French centres of textile production, of Lille, Roubaix and Tourcoing. Belgium had been a major producer of linen cloth and there is evidence that machinery and stock was commandeered and taken to Germany, and many remaining machines destroyed in retaliation for Belgian resistance.

In Britain the Defence of the Realm Act (DORA) drew on thousands of small contractors to meet the demand, such as G. Salamar, who 'owned three inner London workshops that produced clothing for the army',[15] which, incidentally, was a firm engaged to produce the leather jerkins so prized by German officers as a spoil of war. Reserves of cloth were taken up to meet the sudden need for vast quantities of uniform:

> They brought a squad of soldiers to our mill … they'd saved a million yards of cloth from the Boer War … and this squad came with lorries and fetched all this cloth away.[16]

Fabric mills were turned over to the production of khaki fabric. They were thought a fitting outing for a group of recuperating soldiers in their bright blue hospital suits, as if it might cheer them to see that they could soon be back in uniform, one of their number about to return to the trenches recalling the cacophony of industrial machines at full pelt:

> A party was arranged to visit a woollen mill in Bradford … It must have been very interesting but I hadn't heard a word. All those shutters going to and fro.[17]

A vast range of buttons were required by the armed forces, but since many of the factories that had formerly produced them had now been given over to munitions, 'even working shifts around the clock it was many months before the remaining button manufacturers were able to meet the demand'.[18] And since buttons were often what identified one regiment from another, and lower ranks from officers, it was important for morale and a sense of order to keep the men supplied. It is said that the British Army alone commissioned 367 types of button, and that any type of button might be requisitioned within eight hours,[19] – that is ordered, processed and arrived at the trenches within that time.

Fabric Shortages

When materials became scarce, attempts were made to substitute cotton for wool, for example, and there were experiments with artificial fibres to replace silk, as with Piete Kuhr's ersatz fabric blouse (see Chapter 3). In Germany, where cotton was running low, milk proteins were used for a fabric that held dye well, was breathable and able to capture moisture. Unfortunately it also wrinkled too easily, and so required a great deal of ironing after washing. Attempts were made to weave together wool and cotton weft with paper fibre,[20] but it produced a cloth that tended to be too weak for service use. Reclaimed wool mixes were more successful for outer clothing, where its abrasiveness was less of a problem.

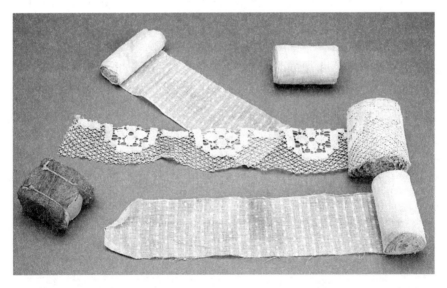

17. Many different materials were used for dressings. The greatest shortages developed in Germany after the Allied naval blockade. Surgical dressing substitutes were made from a range of textiles, including net curtains, and cotton used for petticoats. The most unusual material here (on the left) is sphagnum moss, first used on a large scale by the Japanese during the Russo-Japanese War (1904-5). Sphagnum was an ideal material as it was good for absorbing and keeping hold of liquids, and it had a cooling and soothing effect. Most importantly, sphagnum had antiseptic properties that helped prevent infection and gangrene.

There was also increased production of a cotton-substitute cloth from nettle fibre for German army uniforms. The hollow fibres formed a natural insulation, which could then be twisted if need be, to reduce insulation, making it cool for summer. It was a fabric that had been made for thousands of years, cotton having gained ground only because it had proved easier to harvest and spin. Rayon, known as mother-in-law's silk, had been developed in the second half of the previous century, but it was flammable and expensive, so that little was produced during the war years.[21]

Efforts were made to limit the amount of cloth used domestically. The American government Commercial Economy Board stressed that its efforts to conserve material for the services were designed so that their measures would hardly be noticed by the consumer:

> It has gone to the root and source of clothing supply. It has taken the problem up with the garment manufacturers, the woollen and worsted weavers and the makers of styles … As a result … skirts [will be] a little less full perhaps, fewer patch pockets and belts on men's coats.[22]

For the Central Powers, fabric shortages meant that, even as early as the end of 1914, National Wool Weeks had been instituted, to collect woollen clothing for recycling, sometimes set up as a competition amongst school children as to who could collect the most:

> We have to hand over to the army authorities old jackets, trousers, blankets, shirts, coats and woollens of all kinds. The good materials are made into warm clothing for the soldiers: the inferior materials are pulverised and turned into paper and (I think) material for bandages.[23]

Sister Cecile, the British nun in a Flanders convent who so resented German officers aping Allied pilots (see Chapter 2) again makes her loyalties clear when commenting on spare wool being requisitioned by the German occupation:

> All the wool has to be given in – ours was hidden, and we gave in all the bad wool we had in the house![24]

War was hard on cloth. It wore out, broke down, rotted and disintegrated the carefully chosen fabrics. On both sides of the conflict it was necessary to use the best materials available for combat, keeping shoddier stuff for civilian wear. Fine quality worsted and waterproofed cloth was nonetheless eventually destroyed by the combined assault of weaponry and exposure to the elements.

Not just the fighting men, but the legions of displaced refugees of all ages, cobbling together some protection with whatever pieces of clothing they might find, including stray items of discarded uniform; worn out, desperate POWs, more often the last in any pecking order for care and thus clothing, with ill-treated wounds, feet wrapped in rags, their boots perhaps taken by their captors. Such can be the price of surrender.

In Germany attempts were made to find a substitute for leather soles on boots, since central European leather tended to be too fine for such use. Wooden soles had long been a viable option in rural areas but they were unsuitable for long marches and, for civilian use they were uncomfortable on hard city pavements. Attempts were made to develop a hinged sole to allow more flexibility (as with Piete Kuhr and her classmates in the previous chapter) and finally a flexible metal plate made them a little easier to wear.

There was a measure of organization around salvaged uniform (as suggested in Chapter 2), but the distaste many felt, at the idea of wearing clothes that had once belonged in many cases to the dead, resulted in a certain amount of obfuscation. Local women were employed on both sides of the conflict to recycle and to wash and mend soldiers' clothes, as in the popular soldiers' song 'Mademoiselle from Armentières':[25]

> She got the palm and the *croix de guerre*
> For washin' soldiers' underwear.

Women sorted through discarded clothing collected from the battlefield or from hospital units, some of which, if in reasonable enough condition, was used to uniform the various auxiliary Labour Corps. Allied woollen cloth, too damaged to be mended, was bundled up and regularly sent home to Britain to be turned into blankets, say. For this reason the label 'Pure New Wool' indicated that an item had been made from *un*recycled fibre – and therefore harboured no possibly distressing history of the battlefield.

The Colour of Uniform

Before coming to a decision to wear *Feldgrau*, field grey, for active service uniform cloth, meticulous studies had been undertaken at the turn of the century in Germany, to discover which colours were least easy to spot, comparing grey with khaki and other possibilities:

> The first test was to discover which colour disappeared from sight first. Ten men were dressed, two in dark grey, two in scarlet, two in blue, two in light grey,

and two in green. The first to vanish ... were the pair attired in light grey, and, contrary to all expectations, those dressed in red were the next ... Dark grey, blue, and lastly green, were successively lost to sight ... red was a long way the most difficult colour to hit.[26]

Yet, though red may have passed the test, and red dye would have been an economically viable choice, it was field grey that was adopted. Perhaps the connotations that red has, of anger, danger or even passion, seemed inappropriate, despite its apparent suitability – or more likely it seems that practical considerations of upkeep won out over battlefield safety. Moreover, the 'common sense' notion that red is a bright and noticeable colour, may have held sway despite the evidence of the trials.

The majority of German forces serving in the Ottoman Empire also adopted field grey. Ottoman army officers wore a darker shade of khaki than their men, though this proved an unwise choice in the heat of battle, for enemy snipers could more easily pick them out. The Romanian army adopted uniforms of undyed brown fabric, which came in many shades of grey, green and brown. Bulgarian regiments were insufficiently supplied with German field grey uniforms, and photographs betray their sometimes similarly disparate appearance.

There were rumours that the French army had developed a red, white and blue woven cloth that was practically invisible on the field. After the first months of the war (as discussed in Chapter 2), they too had abandoned their more colourful uniforms. The new, *bleu horizon* cloth, which was thought to be better camouflaged, was a marled pale and darker blue with white flecks. The changeover was of necessity gradual, which meant that certainly for the first years of the war, French troops had a motley appearance. Foreign Legion and Moroccan Infantry corps took on a mustard shade of khaki rather than the horizon blue, a fact most probably explained by the need for sufficient material at short notice, Britain still being a reliable source of khaki cloth.

Khaki had been briefly fashionable in Berlin, known as *Braundrell*, and in Paris and London at the turn of the century, after the South African War, which had

> contributed khaki as a material and as a fashionable colour, khaki hats, blouses and cloth are rampant in the shops, mostly trimmed in red.[27]

Khaki is a term derived from Urdu from the Persian word *khak*, meaning dust. It was first worn by the British Army in India in the late 1840s, after the scarlet tunics and high stocks of the Queen's Own Corps in the Punjab were found to be impractically tight and unsuitable for the climate. Smocks and pyjama trousers were issued in a brown homespun cloth dyed with *mazari* pulp, from a local plant.[28] Belts and boots would not take the dye and so had to be treated with mulberry juice instead, which gives a drab yellowish colour to leather. At the outbreak of the Indian Mutiny in 1857, the regiments raised in the Punjab ran low on *mazari*, so anything that could give a similar hue was used, such as coffee, tea, tobacco and even mud, or a combination of black and red ink. Like German field grey, khaki came to represent the relatively new separation between formal and service dress.

Second only to khaki, the most significant change in the fabric used for British Army uniform was the replacement of leather equipment with canvas or webbing. German and Prussian belts and knapsacks were still being issued in leather even though canvas was lighter, did not corrode bullets and was essentially cheaper to provide. The British new pattern 1908 Web Infantry Belt took over from old leather issue, its multi-functions demonstrated to King George VI:

> The basic equipment consisted of a waist-belt with two cartridge carriers of five pockets each, totalling 150 rounds, from which was hung the bayonet frog and entrenching tool carrier; two 2-inch braces crossed at the wearer's back and passed through diagonally set buckles on the back of the belt; from the bottom ends of these braces were hung the haversack and water bottle. The large pack was carried fastened to the back of the braces, resting in a cradle formed by two cross-supporting straps, so that the load was balanced whether the belt was fastened or not; moreover the whole equipment could be put on and taken off in one piece.[29]

These packs whether of leather or canvas were of a tremendous size and weight when wet, popularly known as the 'Christmas tree'. Soldiers marched with their food, clothing and utensils on their back, a greatcoat rolled up, and perhaps tent poles hanging off with a waterproof haversack containing their personal belongings. During battle they were often left piled up along with anything else that would get in the way of troops being able to move fast:

> Greatcoats had been handed in, tied in bundles of four and, with two hundred thousand packs and three thousand or so officers' valises, were stacked in farm buildings all up and down the line.[30]

Such clothing and accoutrements were often just left to rot, an ominous representation of what became of many soldiers after the Big Push on the Somme.

A long march with a full pack could be punishing:

> I hated that, ten, twelve miles, full pack on my back. Oh well, well ... I used to fall over sometimes ... Twelve to fifteen miles ... rifle weighs about seven or eight pounds, couple of bombs ... blisters all over, army boots all nails, it was a tough time marching.[31]

Cigarettes and other Palliatives

Nonetheless, on a good day, despite his heavy load, Remarque's hero could rejoice in 'the red poppies, the good food, the cigarettes, [and] the summer breeze'.[32] Small luxuries could sustain men living in great discomfort and danger. Cigarettes were associated with leisure, and in the context of war, an aesthetic pleasure that made them for many an essential accessory. They were like clothing, an essential comfort – a small, tactile distraction; a way of separating oneself from the war. For an American trainee pilot far from home, French tobacco was no substitute for American, and 'cigarettes are above all what we need'.[33] The gift of a packet of cigarettes could express sympathy, even solidarity:

> I gave six wounded prisoners a packet of cigarettes ... cannot help but feel sorry for the poor devils.[34]

Men waiting for the order to go over the top would find smoking together a means of steeling their nerve. One young soldier witnessed Saxon troops waving a white flag and then coming to shake hands with British soldiers in no-man's-land, on Christmas Day 1915. The tokens they exchanged were cigarettes, symbolizing their parallel situation: 'They had to do as they were told, same as us.'[35]

If a soldier was to be executed, then it was a common ritual to offer him a cigarette beforehand. In a telling image a cavalryman in the Ottoman army witnesses the death by firing squad of a deserter. The prisoner calmly smokes a cheroot as he is blindfolded and tied to a stake, taking a final draw just as the bullets ring out, one shot pinning his hand to his mouth.[36]

Smoking was not thought of as unhealthy but, on the contrary, as cleansing, warding off bacterial infections and relieving tension, and many photographs exist of recovering soldiers smoking in their hospital beds, even those recovering from gas inhalation, pensively blowing smoke circles from garden chairs in a convalescent home, or on occasion having

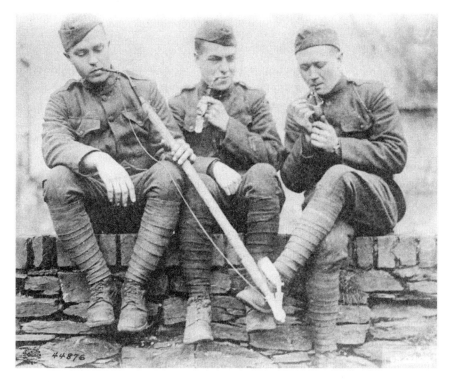

18. Doughboys smoking at Cochem.

their pipes lit by a smiling nurse. Smoking had become more affordable, and 'yellow perils' and 'gaspers' had become a manner of currency for all in trench and field hospital. Even if you did not smoke yourself, a gift of cigarettes or tin of tobacco from the Salvation Army, or the regular issue of, say, two packets of ten and a box of matches once a fortnight, was of value:

> They were horrible things – I couldn't smoke 'em. But you could sell anything, and chaps'd give you 2 francs for one cigarette … and I used to swap my fags for the rum rations.[37]

The tobacco ration, 'like old sailors' twist', that had to be cut up with a knife, was less sought after. As one soldier moves towards the Somme, gradually the cigarettes are used up:

> There was a ration of tobacco and a ration of cigarettes. By the time we got to the front line nobody wanted the hard stuff, so of course a raid was made on the

83

cigarettes. By the time it reached the trenches there was 90% tobacco and 10% cigarettes.[38]

It was still a shocking sight for many to see a woman smoking, intent upon her own private thoughts. A cigarette draws attention to the lips, suggests the pursuit of personal pleasure and possibly a desire to seduce. When women were earning better money, smoking in public, along with eating out, was a sign of new social freedom, when prior to the war this would have been seen as impossibly vulgar, unladylike behaviour, the 'soldier's smoke' or 'the soldier's relief' evidence of female emancipation, 'a visible symbol of defiance and feminism':[39]

A man may take out a woman who smokes for a good time, but he won't marry her, and if he does, he won't stay married.[40]

Some women at work behind the lines took up smoking 'partly to calm their nerves, but mostly to disguise the stench of burning flesh'.[41] However, visiting WAACs in France, a female reporter trusted that these new habits would fail to bring about any fundamental change:

The country will be overrun by cigarette-crazed, mannish, self-opinionated creatures with short hair ... and a distaste for domestic life ... [but] the discipline of army life cannot smother the woman's heart beneath the khaki overcoat, cannot eradicate that homing instinct that is her birthright.[42]

The cigarette could feel like an extension of the body itself – but, when the comfort of nicotine became insufficient, there were age-old consolations of the battlefield. Cocaine and morphine had been available since the mid-nineteenth century in the cities of Europe, from traffic with China and India. Drugs were often in short supply, even amongst the most seriously wounded men, due to transport and communication difficulties. It seems likely that unofficial drug use was more easily available in the port cities of France and Belgium, particularly after the arrival of the Chinese Labour Corps, who were able to set up their own supply lines. Opium was smoked openly for recreation in the Middle East. Amphetamine use was popular in the Turkish lines to counter exhaustion and limited food supplies, supplemented with opium pills and homemade remedies such as Chlorodyne, used in the treatment of cholera, mixed with castor oil.[43]

In the West, non-medical drug use was not necessarily frowned upon as it is today. Department stores on both sides of the conflict marketed gift packets of heroin and cocaine, to send as comforts to men at the front. Moreover, rumours circulated that the authorities, on both sides of the offensive, were secretly dosing their men with bromide in tea, coffee or alcohol, to suppress their sexual drive, but since testosterone can be useful in the field of battle, this seems unlikely.

More than drug use, more even than cigarettes, alcohol was a mainstay for the soldier going into battle, and to be expected to fight without a daily measure of wine, beer or spirit would have felt as difficult for many as fighting without boots or helmet. In the French army cheap wine, *le pinard*, and brandy, *gniole*, was standard issue, and brandy was also doled out daily in the German army.

The tradition in the British army and navy was for rum, one Canadian infantryman describing its use:

> When the front is altogether a beastly place, in fact, we have one consolation. It comes in gallon jars marked simply SRD.[44]

These initials stood for Service Rum Diluted or possibly Special Rations Distribution, though some joked that it should be Seldom Reaches Destination or Soon Runs Dry. Alcohol could motivate men for combat, help them to sleep and even act as a painkiller when drugs were unavailable. Since it was the senior officers who apportioned the alcohol, then its denial could be a means of control and punishment, and the possibility of short measure from a sergeant could keep the men in line, suggesting to them another possible interpretation of SRD: Sergeants Rarely Deliver. For those who acted beyond the call of duty, or carried out particularly distasteful jobs, then an extra measure could be a welcome reward. One young private in the British Army, after the arduous and distressing job of grave digging, welcomed his portion, 'to take the taste of dead men out of my mouth'.[45] On the other hand, doling out too much alcohol could be unwise, making some act rashly, risking their own and their comrades' lives. An officer in the Canadian Corps decided to impose his own teetotal views on his men, handing out tots of fruit juice instead, which earned him the moniker of 'Old Lime Juice'. His senior officer noticed the detrimental effect this had on morale and hastily reinstituted the rum ration.

Given the rigours of their lives, women working in armaments factories, in the Land Army and behind the lines not only took to smoking but also to alcohol, which some put down to the lack of the 'controlling influence' of husband or father. For some it was a habit that was hard to break after the war, though in Britain at least, there is little evidence of any dramatic increase in women's drinking.[46]

Hair

Women were slow to cut off their 'crowning glory', long associated with femininity and erotic promise. Long hair that was neatly restrained in buns might always suggest the possibility of its imminent, intimate release. Long, loose hair could be a liability for women at work. In an image worthy of a mermaid myth, a steward, Violet Constance Jessop, survives being sucked into the rotating propellers of a liner when her rescuers catch sight of the swirling 'vortex of her [long] auburn hair'.[47]

Beverley Nichols suggests that bobs and shingled hair were seen as 'pseudonyms for Sodom and Gomorrah', yet some women delighted in the freedom of shorter hair. They were prepared to take the perceived risk that a haircut might encourage the growth of a moustache or cause baldness, by weakening the 'scalp muscles'.[48] Cutting your hair might entail having to break the news to those back home. Olive King, a driver for the Serbian army, writes to her father that she 'couldn't imagine why [she]'d never done it before'.[49]

However, the view that the war marks a transition in women's attitude to their hair is undercut by the mixed feelings about such innovation at the time. The majority of women continued to wear their hair long, for 'it was as though [women] wanted to be especially feminine out of uniform, for when their men returned from the trenches'.[50] Some compromised by cutting the front short and rolling up the full length of their hair behind. VAD nurses and FANY ambulance drivers, living in conditions sometimes little different from men in the trenches, with very limited washing facilities, nonetheless were disposed to keep their tresses, albeit stinking of sepsis, greasy and infested with lice, fearful of both their mothers' and sweethearts' response if they were to cut them off. Women's hair up until the 1920s was hardly ever cut short.[51]

Those who did cut their hair were not only taking on a more masculine appearance, but also a more masculine sexuality. While shorn hair might suggest the bluestocking intellectual or the nun modestly relinquishing her power to attract, it also could say that she was one of the boys, with the same drives and the same potential availability. On the other hand, Russian female recruits (see Chapters 3 and 5) being marched to a barber's shop and summarily close shaven, were an attempt to produce a 'well-disciplined military unit',[52] and their photographs have an air of the penitentiary, or even of the madhouse.

Short hair for women was perceived as daring, and this connotation still lingers, particularly when women shave their heads entirely, suggesting a challenge to conventional gender roles. When baldness is worn openly today it can also suggest that a woman is undergoing chemotherapy, and not prepared to hide the fact. Some hairdressers at the time kept bottles of smelling salts to hand, to revive clients who might faint when they saw themselves shorn.[53]

For men at war, short hair was generally considered essential, given the limited washing facilities and risk of lice infestation, so that it was usually cut extremely short or shaved off entirely. After nine months on the frontline, a volunteer from New England is happy to have all his hair 'clipped away'. Sikh and some North African troops kept their long hair, but tucked it away in turbans and headdresses and rolled up their beards; some Cossack regiments also kept their hair long, partly plaited, oiled and looped at the side.

While moustaches were widely worn, usually small and neat and sometimes curled, Russian and Balkan troops preferred more abundant mutton-chop sideburns and other styles of facial hair adornment.

Cosmetics

Make-up had been worn surreptitiously by many women since well before the war. Piete Kuhr, in her provincial German town, comments on the older girls at her high school nearly all wearing some, and that her friend Greta does 'very carefully so that the teachers don't notice'.[54] In 1916 one commentator suspects this may be true even of English women:

> Rarely is there seen a faulty complexion in these days. Some may be a little too obviously cared for.[55]

British women on frontline duties received strict orders to avoid 'all powder, paint, scent, earrings or other jewellery etcetera',[56] but such regulations held little sway, when a dab of Guerlain's *L'Heure Bleue* scent or a smudge of rouge was capable of raising the spirits in the often sordid conditions of tent and bivouac. Arnold Bennett remarks in his diaries on the general prevalence of 'painted women' towards the end of the war.[57] *Punch* magazine pictures 'Our Amazon Corps "Standing Easy"' in 1916, all in uniform, all primping and preening, examining their faces in compact mirrors, pouting as they add a little more lipstick here, adjust a kiss curl there.

Many women at work both in the field and at home, with little time one might imagine to dwell on their appearance, nonetheless yearned to assert their femininity. Compact powder, *Bourjois* rouge, sometimes mixed with petroleum jelly or just a little spit to colour the lips, a touch of kohl to frame the eye, and above all mascara – these vanities could circumvent a filthy coal-stained overall or an overcoat heavy with dried mud. Companies

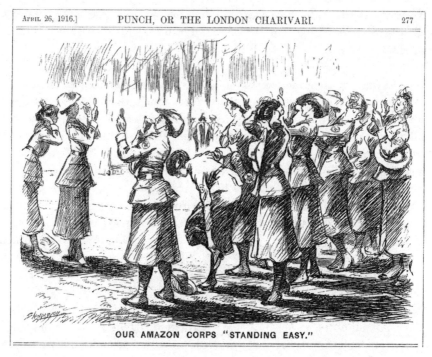

OUR AMAZON CORPS "STANDING EASY."

19. *Punch* cartoon suggesting women continue to consider their appearance, even when in uniform.

like Rimmel and Maybelline, which started up in 1915, made these items affordable – within the economic compass of women of all classes.

Wealthy women, en route to war work – like those who kitted themselves out in high fashion clothing and expensive jewellery to nurse the wounded in France (mentioned in Chapter 3) – did not necessarily want to leave behind their beauty regime. Helena Rubenstein noticed an upsurge in business:

> In London, this specialist's salon is busy packing creams and lotions for Duchesses and ladies, who come in their nurses' uniforms to receive their last complexion instructions before going to the front.[58]

Male use of facial products was still limited, bar some aftershave and proprietary unguents, yet a private on the Somme talks of a perfumier, where 'you could buy Eau de Cologne to mask the unpleasant odour that clung to every uniform and person'.[59] Guerlain's *Jicky* was worn by both men and women of means, its 'clean' scent thought appropriate to wear during the war, plus its non-figurative name allowing men to feel that they were not adopting a flowery, and therefore feminine scent.[60] Hair tonics and oils were more common. *Brillantine,* Brilliantine in Britain, was a popular product to smooth down men's hair, though there was an unfortunate side effect in the trenches, regarding the rat population:

> I was much troubled by them coming and licking the brilliantine off my hair; for this reason I had to give up using grease on my head.[61]

One startling fact is that Romanian army officers below a certain rank were forbidden to wear eye shadow,[62] and indeed this proscription was among the first orders they received at the outset of the war, so that the practice must have been common. Clearly *senior* officers continued to enjoy this privilege, sky blue or lilac lids worn with a monocle perhaps. Norman Stone describes the Romanian army as being particularly reluctant to adopt a drab appearance, and, significantly here, describes them as 'smartly turned out, powdered and painted'.[63]

The Luxury of Being Clean

Cast from the comforts of home, what many longed for was simply the luxury of feeling clean again. Edith Appleton delights in staying at a hotel for the treat of 'bathrooms galore'. One day she finds herself at camp, for once 'quite alone there, and enjoyed it immensely, I bathed, sat with not much on and my hair loose and read'.[64] A bath represented for many the idea of solitary, sensual indulgence.

Dreams of luxurious baths, with steaming hot water, enveloping clean towels and sweet-scented, freshly ironed clothes to put on afterwards, became familiar fantasies for those in factory and trench alike. The young women in Zenna Smith's satire of trench life long for luxurious bathrooms, evoking a sense of opulence in this sumptuous fantasy of bathing

> [with] thick glass shelves loaded with jar upon jar of scented bath salts, white, green, mauve – different colours and different perfumes, lilac, verbena, carnation, lily of the valley. We see ourselves steeped to the neck in over-hot, over-scented water; in our hands are clasped enormous, springy sponges foaming with delicious soapsuds, expensive soapsuds – only the most expensive will suffice – sandalwood, scented oatmeal, odiferous violet. Massage brushes lie to hand, long-handled narrow brushes with quaint, bulbous bristles of hollow rubber that catch the middle of the back just where the arms are too short to reach ... We scrub and scrub and scrub until we are clean and pink and tingling and glowing, we lie in a semi coma until the water begins to cool, but emerging has no terrors.

Electric fires glow softly; before them are spread incredibly huge bath-sheets, soft, lavender-scented, monogrammed, waiting to caress our dripping bodies, to smother them in voluptuous warmth. Now we are dry; we pepper our newly born selves with talcum powder. 'June Roses' fills the air with its fragrance, daintily argues with the scent of the bath water, triumphs.[65]

The detail here implies the contrasting reality of their everyday lives in a tented camp – of cold water in limited supply, of mean facilities, of cold and stench and exhaustion. For one soldier, lying in hospital suffering from trench fever but clean at last, he could feel safe from the miseries of Ypres, 'as near to heaven as I could hope to be'.[66] If the wound were not too severe, hospital meant the chance of feeling cosseted:

We took in the scene with hungry and glaring eyes – ACTUAL BEDS with clean sheets, most of them occupied with clean-shaven men, cleanliness everywhere … [I] lay on my back and breathed long and deep, exquisite was the feel of clean linen.[67]

Central Powers and Allied troops fighting on the Eastern Front might sometimes enjoy the luxury of a Turkish bath. These were at first out of bounds to British soldiers, but for one lieutenant, who had been camping out without tents or blankets with clothes freezing hard to his skin, his filthy state had begun to seem like a form of protection. He recalls stripping away his clothes and fearing that he was now naked to the enemy.[68]

A steaming hot bath in the nearest hotel may have been the first thing many wanted on leave, but, belying any need for privacy, baths were sometimes managed behind the lines. Imagine a makeshift bathhouse set up on the Western Front in an old brewery barn, in the manner of bravura comedy:

Each man carrying his underclothes under an arm, they hopped, naked and crooked and tense in the cold air, playing jokes on one another, to the shed where they handed over the smelly woollen bundles. Then clutching their grey, soiled little towels, they loped with exaggerated shivering into the cavernous room where stood the mash tubs … Six men to a steaming tub … Pass the soap, Ginger, 'strewth, … crikey what a pair … The sinking water was sucked away … and ogh! Cold gushed out of the tap.[69]

Portrayals of soldiers bathing together are common in accounts of the war, showing the human body at its most defenceless. Men are photographed in underwear trooping to a bathhouse, or bathing in a river, enjoying a rare opportunity to be clean. Their nakedness betrays both their fleshly vulnerability and also their shared humanity, stripped of rank and sign of allegiance. Before the battle of the Somme, Siegfried Sassoon describes 'how young and light-hearted' the men look, bathing in the open. Edmund Blunden imagines the Germans being happy to turn a blind eye to a party of Tommies who 'splashed and plunged yards from enemy lines'.[70] A British soldier describes some of his fellows taking a shower by the Somme, and having to run for their lives. Somehow the fact that they are wearing their boots alone makes them seem both comic and touching. They need clothes not just for protection but because they cease to be soldiers without them:

> Chaps came running out in only their shoes, boots on, nothing else on ... so when they finished shelling we had to go to the quarter bloke to get clothes for them.[71]

When a party of exhausted Russian prisoners first arrives, Gaston Riou describes how he and other French POWs take on their care, expressed here as if they were mothers with their helpless babies:

> A tribe of naked little fathers ... How thin they were! Smiling, making awkward little gestures, each one of them allows himself to be manipulated by a Frenchman, who soaped him all over, rubbed him down, pummelled him, dried him, and finally dressed him.[72]

Months earlier the same diarist had described the joy of taking a bath after being taken captive, expressed in the language of sensual transport, delighting in being free of his uniform. It is as if in being naked he surrenders:

> Oh that first *teube*! [bath] After I had worn my clothes continuously for so many days and nights ... the forbidden and unhoped for sensation, to be, as if at home, naked beneath the steaming water; the lather of soap everywhere, on the hair, the neck, the chest, the arms, the legs, the feet; the douche and the aid of a bailer; the dry rub! At length to have a clean skin and clean linen! ... I am clean; what a luxury! I am in their hands but I have managed to get clean ... I am a prisoner; but I have secretly divested myself of my coating of filth, a burden almost as heavy as hunger![73]

A German officer, in a letter to his parents, describes in heightened, romantic terms – almost as if it were some richly coloured medieval tapestry – coming across a body of men bathing near Lodz:

Today we rode along by the Bzura to bathe. At the old bullet-ridden mill we suddenly came upon a gleaming medley of naked, glittering bodies of men and horses; there were shouts and cries and a gorgeous game of mirth and laughter. Quickly we undressed and rode our horses into the water. A gorgeous blue sky, a thronging mass of naked people.[74]

There was little provision made for washing yourself or your clothes in the frontline, where any supply of water had to be either carried in or collected from shell holes. If a mug of water were spared for shaving, then half a dozen men might be expected to make use of it.[75] When an opportunity does occur for a soldier to enjoy a shave in private, an officer is quick to share the pleasure:

I just lathered up and the sun was shining in this particular day ... I had a small mirror stuck into this bit of ground at the side of the sniping post ... I had a lovely shave, and my platoon officer came round and he said, 'Oh, what a clean boy!' I didn't have a lot of growth in these days, but I had a lot of whiskers, and he remarked about my ability in handling a razor, you see ... 'cause it was then

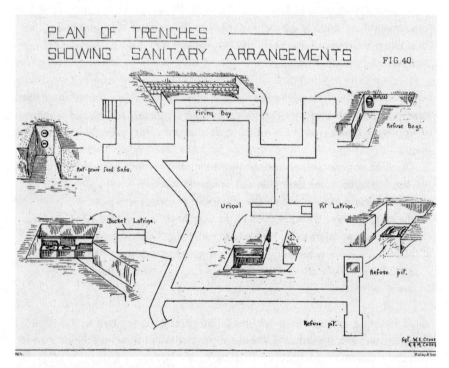

20. A lantern slide showing sanitary arrangements in the trenches, c.1918.

that the safety razor had just come out and nearly everybody used a cut-throat, but there was cuts all over the place ... kept on nicking themselves ... So, he wanted one [a shave] too. I said 'You sit down there, sir. I'll give you a shave, sir.' I shaved him.[76]

For a man accustomed to feeling clean-shaven, such rare moments could be important. Shaving is associated with a sense of manly maturity; older 'career' soldiers, the 'old sweats', dubbed young volunteers 'smoothies', their lack of whiskers suggesting they were still children, and thus of less use as warriors. Safety razors had been around since the turn of the century, but they were seldom available to the troops on either side of the conflict, and even the cut-throat variety could be in short supply and open to pilfering. A private voices his company's suspicions:

When we were on the Somme ... we had the French cavalry there. We'd only have to put our shaving gear down for a minute or two to get a towel or whatever, by the time you got back to pick up your razor it had gone ... We always blamed these line fellows of the French cavalry. Very good at pinching razors![77]

The Gillette disposable was included in American field kits from 1917, and was so appreciated that by the end of the war troops were allowed to keep their razors as a valued perk. Contact with the new safety razors meant that many different nationalities went home determined to get one for themselves.

The majority of women did not shave their legs before the war, and indeed bodily hair was considered erotic, armpit hair in particular, suggesting other more hidden parts. Shorter skirts and finer stockings meant leg hair began to be seen as unattractive. *Harper's Bazar*, an up-market American women's magazine, carried an advertisement in 1915 showing a model in evening gown with armpits on display, smooth as a ten-year-old girl's – though it was not until the sleeveless dresses of the 1920s that women took to shaving their armpits. Gillette introduced *Milady Décolletée* razors in 1915, prettily boxed for the fashion conscious; body hair for women in much of the West, including excess facial hair and pubic hair, was beginning to be seen as both unhygienic and ultimately unfeminine.[78]

Underwear

What lay beneath a uniform could be as important as its outward appearance, in terms of comfort and morale. When the Australian Corps reached France they found that there was little provision for bathing or laundry. While stocks allowed they could exchange dirty clothing for clean, but there was seldom enough to go around. Though each man was meant to carry at least one spare pair of underpants and two pairs of socks, these were soon used up. Sometimes men had to survive for weeks without:

> I well remember our pleasure on being marched to the Outhersteene Baths on the warm afternoon of the 26th to find that there was a certain amount of clean under clothing there for us. It had been washed at the adjoining Laundry by French and Belgian women ... From then until September, however, we heard no more of Baths or clean clothing in the 4th Division.[79]

Ordinance Corps had to arrange for dirty clothing to be disinfected and deloused, and negotiate the use of hotel washing machines, but even then there were major difficulties in drying vast amounts of clothing in the winter months. Various drying rooms were attempted, with cables and cross wires, and later with fans. Moreover, each time a company moved, advancing and retreating often over the same territory, then new arrangements had to be made.

Women joining the Russian Battalion of Death were issued with warm woollen underwear, which would have been an unheard of luxury for most before the war. In the WAAC in Britain, which sought to appeal to a wider class of women, the regulations stated that you should provide your own underwear, but it was soon noticed that many poorer recruits came without any experience of underwear whatsoever, as 'knickers were an upmarket item'.[80] Knickers thus became standard issue for women's service uniforms, though sometimes the size was not considered important, one ATS recruit complaining about their fit, mirroring a similar problem for male soldiers issued with clean underwear (see Chapter 2):

> If they hadn't got your size you were issued with whatever size they had. I had a pair of khaki silk bloomers that I could hold under my chin, and they reached below my knees.[81]

The First World War did not do away with corsets altogether, despite accounts to the contrary. However, it has been said that the war dealt 'a moral blow to the corset and increases the popularity of the bra'.[82] Many older women continued to wear what they had always worn, choices for the unfashionable always lagging behind youthful daring. Many wore stays to make them look slimmer, and on the Allied side, women were discouraged from leaving off their corsets by propaganda suggesting that German women were fat and frumpy.

For those who kept on their corsets, the need for armament materials meant that non-metal stays, such as those made of Coralene, were more widely adopted.[83] Paul Poiret had used more supple girdles from as early as the 1900s in Paris, but they were still very constricting, and not necessarily more comfortable, but at least they looked as if they were. The body was no longer – amongst the fashionable at least – held rigidly in place. Advances in the manufacture of rubberized elastic material in 1911 made the new longer line girdles more wearable, with Chanel recommending more comfortable underpinnings to allow a softer line. Valerie Steele points out that the French fashion designer Madeleine Vionnet insisted that it was she, and she alone, who had single-handedly got rid of the need for a corset with her bias-cut designs.

Comfortable corsets advertised for those of more moderate income include the new 'Free Hip Bone' style, promising comfort for the fuller figure and the 'Side Spring' offering 'perfect freedom to the wearer'.[84] Elasticated girdles were believed to have comparable beneficial effects on the body, and yet provide a more natural looking silhouette than what came before. Others declared that a soft bodice alone was best for women's health and comfort and that a lack of restriction would allow the body to find its 'natural' proportions. For women with fuller breasts this was unconvincing advice, and bodices were designed to support and shape them, the beginnings of the modern support brassiere.

Florence Nightingale had banned her nurses from wearing corsets in the mid-nineteenth century, but many found the old ways of dressing so familiar that they were slow to relinquish them. If your back was accustomed to artificial support, then it could be uncomfortable to do without. Corsets were believed to support the inner organs. It was moreover an unnerving sensation to have your breasts separated and supported by straps from above, rather than squeezed together and raised from below. Partly because of the lack of availability of bras, and their expense, many young women left off corsets to wear just bloomers and woollen or cotton jersey vests, combinations, or buttoned bodices.

Petticoats, which had long been associated with femininity, seemed out of kilter with the new practical woman. Yet many seemed still to yearn for lace, and the suggestiveness of a petticoat that peeps below a hemline. It was not only the highly fashionable woman in the new *Kriegskrinoline* or Parisian silhouette, but also uniform skirts adapted to allow more freedom of movement that provided an opportunity for the frivolity of the petticoat to return. Inversely, just as long-legged knickers had come about to wear under the original crinolines, wide-legged silk and cotton knickers made it more comfortable to wear full unlined woollen skirts, avoiding the need for an abundance of petticoat.

German service underwear was rumoured to be better made and of more serviceable quality than Allied. The British government was determined to discover exactly what it was that they were wearing. It was not only a question of keeping the men warm, but of finding clothing that would not chafe in damp conditions. British officers were ordered to collect samples of enemy underwear from the dead, to be assessed for quality and design in the freezing winter of 1914:

> We were requested to send back specimens of German army under-clothing. Paige and Babbage, most mild of garden-loving men, have to cut the clothing off with jack-knives. The frost has made it particularly difficult.[85]

What the German troops turned out to be wearing was varied, some issued with separate vests, with long or short sleeves depending on the weather conditions, and underpants, with legs to the knee or sometimes right down to the ankle. Summer or tropical issue would be of cotton, and sometimes a lighter weight vest of cotton string, or woven with a pattern of holes; wool the warmest option for cold weather. Although the British upper classes had enjoyed patented Aertex vests, on very similar lines to the German fine string vests, since the late nineteenth century, they were not available to ordinary serviceman,[86] worn only by the officer class if they so chose. One-piece combinations became popular, influenced by American union suits, which avoided the gap at the waist of two-piece underwear.

Souvenirs

It is normal, even in war, to want to find gifts to send back home. Partly presents restore normality in extraordinary circumstances, as if the sender is merely on holiday, having a good time, soon to return with all her or his stories. American pilot Allen Peck, for example, bought his sweetheart a pair of high heels on a visit to Paris, and Clarence Bush, an American artilleryman, sent home powder compacts to each of his three sisters. Wristwatches were often given to men, since pocket watches were impractical in the trenches. Previously they had been worn by women alone, but during the war they became a useful, if expensive present, worn on the inside of the wrist to protect the glass face – a practice continued by some ex-military men today.

Gifts made in the trenches could also remind those at home that the giver was at war, and the materials harvested from the field of battle, though often disguised, gently brought this home. Sometimes troops passed the long hours of waiting by taking up a hobby of embroidery, carpentry or carving perhaps, using whatever materials were to hand. Hawkers would sell their wares to troops, fashioned with ingenuity from the leftovers of war: spent shells, bullets, fuses, wire, splintered wood and bone, scavenged from the field. Would an ornament made from a segment of metal shell or a crucifix carved from a fragment of wood, not harbour some intention to show what these men were facing, of live shells falling and of the splintered bones of their companions? The wide variety of items, made or purchased, with a direct reference to the conflict are known as trench art.

Souvenirs were usually patriotic in theme, and often highly sentimental. A homesick nurse might send home an ornamental pillowcase embroidered *Von einem liebende Tochter* (From a Loving Daughter) to reassure her parents that she was still their own, despite her newfound independence. The word that appears again and again in these artefacts is Mother, *Mutter, Maman, Madre, Majka, Mor ...*

Jane Kimball describes POWs making trench art to raise money, enough for much needed food and small luxuries such as cigarettes. The civilian internment camp of Ruhleben near Berlin would hold exhibitions of their wear, from reworked silver coin to wallets sewn from rat skins. Charles Grauss, garrisoned in France, carved a set of wooden animals to send home to his little girl, Ghislaine, accompanied by a letter showing in cartoon form how one day he planned to build a beautiful house for his family. He was

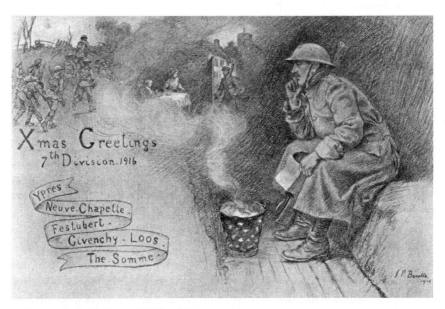

21. Christmas in the trenches and thinking of home.

never, in fact, to make it home, killed in action in April 1918.[87] Convalescent troops were given craftwork to help speed their recovery, perhaps to take their minds off disabling injuries or to help alleviate the symptoms of mental distress that became known as shell shock.

Women concerning themselves with jewellery could seem too frivolous as the war progressed, so that wearing bibelots that could be justified in terms of their patriotic origin became fashionable. So-called sweetheart jewellery was often made in the form of a heart, or clasped hands, playing on the bond between soldiers and their home. Trench jewellery whether made by soldiers, civilians or commercial enterprise, expressed patriotism and bore a certain piquant allure on account of its association with the battlefield. Marcel Proust noticed the prevalence of military style jewellery on the boulevards of Paris, 'the fashion now was for rings or bracelets made out of fragments of exploded shells or copper bands from 75mm ammunitions',[88] matched by the craze for military designs in women's civilian wear (discussed in Chapter 3).

A cheap, sentimental gift bought on leave for a girlfriend, perhaps from a fairground stall, might be as inexpensive as a little kewpie doll, named after Cupid, with rosy cheeks and a little curl right in the middle of its forehead. The design, patented in 1913, was taken from the illustrations of Rose O'Neill in the *Ladies Home Journal* of 1909, but manufactured in Ohrdruf, Germany, a centre for toy manufacture. It was first produced in bisque but later in cheaper materials such as celluloid, wood and paper, and was made in France and Belgium after the outbreak of war. The image was so popular that some women plucked their eyebrows in a thin high arch to resemble the dolls. Kewpies were also used for high-end gold jewellery during the war, combining kitsch with conspicuous expense. Silver was more affordable, un-rationed because it was not required for arms' manufacture.

Mizpah jewellery, popular from the late nineteenth century but enjoying a revival during the war, derived from a biblical idea of there being a lasting connection between people who are apart, even after death: 'The Lord watch between me and thee this day, when we are absent one from another'.[89] It is sometimes made from gold or silver, incorporating images of the Bible or combined hearts, perhaps entwined with ivy, and often with the word *mizpah* as an integral part of the design. A ring or brooch might be sent home to Germany or a Parisian wife might purchase a tiepin for a husband to wish him safe return.

In all the uncertainties of war, with families separated and lives disrupted, there was perhaps something reassuring in these small totems of affection. Moreover, whether the gift be a cheap kewpie doll, a gold angel *mizpah* locket or a fashion doll bought at great expense in Paris for your girlfriend back home, all might be seen as cute representations of the body, and as a relief from the reality of the brutal disfigurements of the war. A small point of xenophobia here is that German doll heads already in stock in Paris at the beginning of the war had their marks of origin removed before sale, as a patriotic duty.[90] A doll might be a romantic or sentimental gesture, an escape from the war, but it should not ignore which side was which.

Official gifts acted as formal acknowledgement of a soldier's sacrifice. The Kaiser sent Christmas presents of cigars in the first year of the conflict, ten for each soldier, in a box inscribed: '*Weinachten im Feld 1914*' (Christmas in the field 1914).[91] The public were encouraged to send parcels to the men, known as *Weinachtspakaten* (Christmas parcels) or *Liebepaketen* (love parcels). Piete Kuhr helps with packing up parcels for the front, her favourite novelty item underlying the importance of cheerful items that nonetheless had a practical purpose:

> The nicest presents were thirteen little puppets. They consisted of a large pink handkerchief which was sewn on to a body with coarse stitches. The head was filled with sweets. Three bath sponges formed the hair, nose and beard; the eyes were buttons. The arms and legs were stuffed with a cigar, the body filled with a packet of tobacco. Instead of a rifle the soldier-puppet had a pipe under his arm. The knapsack was a reel of thread with a needle stuck in it.[92]

The magazine *La Vie Parisienne* encouraged readers to send parcels to soldiers as *marraines de guerre* (wartime godmothers) containing foodstuffs and small items of clothing. Men might be 'adopted' by several of these *marraines*, one French soldier recalling:

> One of my *marraines* sent me flowers, perfume, cigars and a stocking to make a scarf of. That was a very nice souvenir.[93]

Tins sent out to British troops, as a 'gift from the nation' in the name of Princess Mary, were often kept long after the contents had been consumed. They were initially made of brass, though after the sinking of the Lusitania, when a large order of brass was lost at sea, they came to be made of poorer quality alloys. The lids of these tins were embossed with the head of the 17-year-old princess, and with the names of all the Allied countries: Belgium, France, Britain, Montenegro, Serbia, Russia and Japan. Inside the contents varied, from an ounce of tobacco and cigarettes in yellow monogrammed wrappers, pipe and lighter, to pencils and packets of sweets for non-smokers. Indian troops were given sweets and spices, whereas nurses were often sent chocolates. A sergeant has little use for the cigarettes he receives and gives them to his friends, but the tin comes in useful for protecting the Bible his mother had given him when he signed up:

> It fitted the box perfectly. That's the only thing I brought home from the war.[94]

Many were anxious to find souvenirs, taking risks to attain them. One British private at Passchendaele noted this sometimes reckless urge, as if the pickings could compensate them for the trenches. The dead enemy became a resource:

> There were some chaps in our lot who would do anything for souvenirs, so, while we were waiting for the barrage to lift, they got out of the trench and started searching these bodies for anything they could get. They were after watches and buttons and things like that.[95]

A British soldier about to take his first leave from the front, decides to create a souvenir with a story:

> [I] took off my hat [steel helmets weren't invented then] put it on the bankside and put a bullet through it. I did it so that when I went home wearing a hat with a bullet hole through it, I could say, 'That was a near one!' And that's what I did.[96]

One of the most sought after presents and souvenirs was enemy headgear. Richard Harding describes soldiers searching enemy trenches 'intent only on finding a spiked helmet … They were as happy and eager as children picking wild flowers'.[97] *Pickelhauben*, spiked helmets, were the most desirable 'because of their brass eagles surmounted with the inscription "*Gott Mit Uns*"', God with us. In 1918 a group of Canadian soldiers was photographed emerging from a cellar in Cambrai with an armful of them following the city's capture in October 1918. These finds could later be decorated with flowers, romantic messages and sometimes flags. Alison Lurie makes the general point that the stiffer the hat the more status they tend to carry,[98] comparing soft caps with bowler or top hats, say. In this context the *Pickelhaube*, with its rigid uncompromising height, is emasculated by such pretty decoration and its use as a present or memento reinforces Allied domination.

Clarence Bush, the American airman, writes that he hopes to secure German prisoner of war caps, 'as souvenirs, and also caps from the French. I am trying to get one each for myself'.[99]

Sometimes souvenirs could be troubling. An Australian soldier took home a Turkish human head from the Gallipoli campaign, found many years later in mummified form, though the fact that it was stored in a velvet-lined box perhaps suggests that the resonance of such a body part was not overlooked. A German officer considers making a souvenir of a macabre find, attempting a wry objectivity, yet he decides to leave it be:

> This afternoon I found two fingers still attached to the metacarpal bone near the latrine of the Altenburg fortress. I picked them up and had the tasteful idea of having them worked into a cigarette holder. But there was still greenish-white decomposed flesh between the joints ... so I decided not to.[100]

Despite the prevalence of such disturbing mementos in wartime, there was a desire to associate collecting body parts, say, as something other, that a more Western-orientated soldier would not choose to do. There are accounts, for example, of Senegali *Tirailleurs* collecting body parts, like anthropological surveys of primitive behaviour:

> They take few prisoners and have a fancy for the ears, fingers and even the heads of their victims. The ears and fingers are threaded on string and form a gruesome necklace while the heads are carried in a *musette* till the odors from them leads to their discovery.[101]

And yet, not everyone sought mementos of the conflict. A British soldier offered the piece of shrapnel that has been extracted, without anaesthetic, from his groin, retorts:

> Souvenir? I've had the bloody thing too long already. Throw it away![102]

Some took a generally unsentimental view:

> I don't want no souvenirs ... They gone barmy over souvenirs. What are you doing with souvenirs if you don't know you're going to get back or not ... I wouldn't have anything to do with anything like that.[103]

Instant Images

Photography had become much more affordable. The Box Brownie camera had been on the market since 1900 and was light and compact enough to mean that amateur photographers with the wherewithal could take photographs more easily even in the field of battle. Max Arthur remarks that photographs of enemy corpses were popular trophies in the German lines.[104]

For many though a studio photograph, taken before men went off to fight or while on leave, was what was wanted as a keepsake. We see the young recruit, newly shaven in his khaki or field grey; later the grainy images taken in the line, now in worn uniform, he stares dazed into the camera lens with his tunic loose and torn, his puttees half undone; a group of men are caught laughing, German troops in their newly acquired British fur jerkins; British soldiers 'peacocking about in German helmets, taken with their own hands and proudly showing their souvenirs'.[105] These moments are caught on camera.

Photography businesses flourished in the lines, making it possible to send back a portrait as a gift with little delay. A young British rifleman writes home with a photograph of himself in his new uniform:

> I was taken at 5.00 and they were ready at 7.15, so you can see it was sharp work. They only cost 1/- for the half dozen.[106]

***

For many the experience of the conflict made even the most ordinary items seem transformed, or rather as the months drew on, what had seemed normal became touched by the confusions of war. One might not want to collect souvenirs, but this did not mean these items, their fabric, substance and resonance, were not felt. An American nurse quietly expresses her sense of this incongruity when a man's brains could come away in her hand as bandages are undone and at the same time a discussion is going on between the surgeons – about where to eat the best oysters. The scent of this normality is disinfectant, *eau de javel* [bleach], iodoform and the swamp gas stench of gangrene. The world has become the war:

> My clothes hanging on pegs, my white aprons and rubber boots ... the big sharp scissors on the table – all these familiar things are touched with magic and make me uneasy ... There is wet mud on my boots and blood on my apron.[107]

5 ATTITUDES TO THE BODY

All that is associated with dress, its accessories and accoutrements, its points of style – all, I have suggested, contribute to our understanding of the First World War, and of the individuals that lived through that period. Clothing covers the body. It flatters, protects, enhances and sometimes betrays what lies beneath. The body then, and the extent to which it was exposed, hidden, gained sexual experience say, suffered venereal disease, craved drugs, was subject to injury or simply how it was lived in, is part of this story. The body lies in curious relation to our sense of self. It is both something we feel we own but is also what we cannot exist without. Jonathan Miller refers to the body as 'a large part of what we actually are'.[1] One speaks figuratively of the body of an army, the body of a nation, but ultimately it is individual flesh and blood humanity on which war relies.

National Identity and the Mother Goddess

Before looking at attitudes to the body in particular individuals, I want to consider how the warring nations saw themselves. The ways in which different nationalities were embodied affected how individuals saw themselves in relation to the war and how loyalty and enmity were established. Marianne, the personification of the French nation is depicted as both nursing mother[2] and fearsome warrior, wearing a Phrygian cap, symbol of a revolution;[3] Britannia is strong and womanly with shield, centurion's helmet and trident, sometimes flanked by a lion, as symbol of natural power. Mother Russia is portrayed on a poster in 1914 standing between Marianne and Britannia, all three in flowing classical robes. Germany is the *Heimatland*, or Germanic Homeland, known as *Vaterland*, or Fatherland – so male, yet from the early nineteenth century there is also the female *Germania*, warrior Rhine maiden, and it is this image that re-emerged with a vengeance in 1915. In Friedrich August von Kaulbach's painting *Deutschland August 1914*, Germania is a sensual figure with flaming hair, wearing breastplate, a helmet crown and carrying both sword and shield.

All these female images of nationhood suggest full-bodied womanliness, dressed in costumes reminiscent of the Art Nouveau movement, of sinuous silk, lace and brocade *Merveilleuses* dresses at the Longchamps races before the war, rather than war workers in practical, got up uniforms. It is the fashion of the archetype, the goddess watching over and nurturing, and sometimes forcefully motivating the world of mere men, manifestations of 'The hand that rocks the cradle is the hand that rules the world'.[4]

Propaganda images, more often in poster form, were employed by all sides, sometimes straightforward in their message but in others with a degree of sophistication. Looking at how these images are represented, and in particular how their bodies are dressed, soldiers shown in tattered clothing are intended to garner sympathy; women in sexually suggestive clothing are to evince moral distaste and remind what women should be. Joan of Arc offers a more subtle form of persuasion, in the opposition between her vulnerable female body and the carapace of male armour; France is later depicted with full chest and wide hips, but now in breeches, victorious above the wasteland of the trenches.

Nurses on posters are more often shown as maternal, and the wounded men they watch over are thus their children. Though Allied propaganda might show a German nurse cruelly pouring water on the ground in front of a thirsty wounded British soldier,[5] German posters depict nurses in full-length uniforms with nun-like wimples and eyes modestly cast down.[6] In a British design, a nurse is shown *pietà*-like – as the Virgin Mary with a soldier as the Christ figure, bandaged and leaning on a crutch to one side, and to her other a small child clings to her skirts as she shields it from harm, as if to confirm her role as blessed mother.[7]

Those far from home might dwell on thoughts of their own mothers, or the idealized notion of motherliness at least, longing for a time when it would be possible to feel safe and be treated as an individual again.

If it is men who are the fodder of warfare – civilian casualties aside – then it is women who are presented as the providers of men, devoted or tyrannical, matriarch or siren, encouraging and motivating its transport. The poet Alfred Noyes describes women of the munitions factories as 'motherly', as if the shells produced were their tender offspring. Wilfred Owen has a hospital barge suggesting a pregnant woman, the boat passing through a lock in 'bulging amplitude', so that one might imagine the wounded soldiers returned to the womb.[8] In a letter home he compares no-man's-land with an infected human body, 'pot-marked like a body of foulest disease and its odour is the breath of cancer'.[9] Just as single female figures stand for the pregnant and proliferating war, the war comes to embody individual humanity.

In this context, Zenna Smith depicts women as indifferent to suffering, with those at home described as 'ever-knitting women safe from the blood and mud'.[10] Virginia Woolf satirizes those who 'used all their immense stores of charm ... to persuade young men that to fight was heroic'.[11]

Officers in the field sometimes took on what could be seen as a maternal role towards their men, in the sense that they came to care for their physical and emotional needs, and this relationship was often mutual:

> One of the paradoxes of the war – one of the many – was that this most brutal of conflicts should set up a relationship between officers and men that was ... domestic. Caring ... maternal ... The war that had promised so much in the way of 'manly' activity had actually delivered 'feminine' passivity, and on a scale that their mothers and sisters had scarcely known.[12]

Batmen

One might argue further that women failed in their maternal role by sending men to war. In the stalemate of a war of attrition, any easy delineation between mother figure as facilitator and father figure as rule-maker broke down. The conditions of trench warfare in particular meant men were effectively trapped together at close quarters for long periods of inactivity, in the knowledge that at any moment they might be attacked or be required to attack. The exchange of care between officers and their men, between batmen and their charges, allowed a degree of intimacy that civilian life often had not. Home meant the old order of relations between the sexes; the First World War in this sense interrogated former gender relations.

Their personal servants, or batmen, took on their officers' domestic care, which one might typify as a maternal, or at least as a parental role. Pat Barker's fictive version of the psychiatrist, Dr Rivers, treating shell-shocked soldiers at Craiglockhart War Hospital in Scotland 1917, questions the notion that a caring attitude should necessarily be associated with women:

> The implication that nurturing, even when done by a man, remains female, as if the ability were in some way borrowed, or even stolen, from women.[13]

Far from the firing line, officer and servant were less intimately engaged. One bookish upper middle-class man found himself deemed unsuitable officer material, and was thrown into a new existence as a batman in the

British Royal Flying Corps. Despite his initial unwillingness to take on what he considers a demeaning role, he finds himself taking pride in keeping his officer's boots clean:

> With the aid of brown Kiwi polish and Soldier's Friend, polishing rags and an old toothbrush for the buttons, using your button stick, of course, and spitting into the tin of Soldier's Friend.[14]

However, despite his best efforts, the boots are never clean enough. He makes too much noise tiptoeing into the officer's room with morning tea, and consequently has to suffer the indignity of wearing tennis shoes comically too large. But this is all part of a batman's life, as the poor man comes to acknowledge:

> A batman himself is a subject of joking, when one comes to think of it, although he may not always see the point of the jest.[15]

In the close confines of trench life the relationship could become highly charged. Graham Seton of the Inverness-shires, tells the tale of his own young batman, Peter, in highly sentimental terms, using the language of romance. He is described as 'roughly tender and bravely beautiful', as if the foundling Glaswegian is his child, parent or perhaps lover, 'the best and most intimate friend man ever had'.[16] Peter makes sure his officer's uniform is cleaned and mended. He learns to insert a fork heated in a brazier into the pleats of a kilt to drag out the lice,[17] and keeps Seton supplied with tobacco at all times. As with a mother raising her offspring, no aspect of the officer's personal comfort is out of bounds.

When Seton returns home on leave to the Surrey hills, he takes Peter with him, 'to the luxury of white sheets, bright firesides, warm baths and the mellow quietness of warm hearts'.[18] The young man entertains the family, playing the bagpipes, taking a subordinate role again. As with all the best sentimental memoirs, when Seton writes about his 'faithful servant, a friend and counsellor, an ever-present companion to give me confidence in the darkness of a dangerous night, and good cheer',[19] he is writing about someone buried in the past, in Ration Farm Cemetery near La Chapelle.

Gaston Riou, POW in a German fortress, happily accepts one of a group of Russian prisoners as his servant, as if, like the care of an assiduous mother, the man would not have taken no for an answer:

> He polishes my shoes … he brings me water for my 'teube' [bath] … if the cloth of my worn trousers, too skimpy for me … gives way during an unusually

vigorous movement of Swedish gymnastics; he promptly threads a needle and repairs the damage; he watches over me as one watches milk on the boil; no valet ever served me so well.[20]

The relationship was not always so easily accommodated. A young German officer has reservations about allowing another man to play so intimate, and as he sees it, inferior a part in his domestic life:

> Batmen are a bit of a problem. I do not see at all why I should be superior to men who are just as good or better than myself in all the qualities needed here … That is why I do not like having my stirrups polished by a man who, in experience, knowledge and capacity, is my superior, and with whom I feel on an equal footing.[21]

Androgynous Bodies

Just as war allowed men to interact with each other away from women's critical eye, women too had opportunity to be relatively free from male judgement. In relation to clothing, when the corset was left off for example, it revealed a more 'masculine' body shape, particularly for those reared on women with rigid S-bend figures. Male and female bodies were found surprisingly alike, give or take. Moreover, their clothing and behaviour had become less delineated. Women going about in trousers, masculine overcoats, socks and boots, even shorn hair and smoking and driving trucks, appeared as if they did not care how they were seen. In counterpoint, men were immobilized in this war of attrition. They wore tatty uniforms, came home on leave filthy, lousy and discouraged. When they did fight their bodies were no match for modern weaponry, ripped open, with no glorious death but left to rot on a battlefield, as food for rats. When they survived they did not always return as they had once been, scarred and disabled but also with minds impaired, in mute shock, in angry disintegration. The modern man at war had little to do with the soberly dressed, sober mien of the late nineteenth- and early twentieth-century gentleman:

> In the thickness of material and solidity of structure of their tailored garments, and in the heavy and sober blackness of their shoes, in the virgin whiteness and starched stiffness of their collars and of their shirt fronts, men exhibit to the outer world their would-be strength, steadfastness and immunity from frivolous distraction.[22]

It must have been bewildering for men to lose this sense of gravitas. When they signed up they were stripped of clothing that once had given them a sense of their place in the world. And when uniforms were provided, they were not the magical warrior garments of the past. Clothing was often ill designed for the conditions in which they found themselves, but at least it was the same for their fellows, and common suffering bred comradeship.

There was little privacy in the field. In this sense the body was more exposed. Cleanliness and previous habits of modesty were difficult to maintain. You might, for example, have no alternative but to relieve yourself in public:

> Twelve to a tent they slept; there was no privacy. John Bullock was still shy about the outer functions of his body, and was unable to squat with the others on the latrines, which were dug close together near the washing place, a hundred dog-graves in the turf, and open to the sky. He used to wait until darkness, and then, if it were not too late, he would seek his own privy far from the camp and meditate upon the strangeness of the world.[23]

This is hardly to suggest that privacy had been enjoyed by all prior to the war. Privies may not have been communal, but many of the poor would have lived in cramped and unhygienic conditions.

Sexual Mores

One area of changing attitudes to the body lies in relation to sexual matters. The war brought about a greater knowledge and use of contraception and prophylactics. There were new opportunities for sexual adventure, not only for men, but also, in their absence, women too were able to question previously prescribed roles.

Venereal disease was a near inevitable consequence of greater sexual freedom, though, as the war progressed, some came to see a dose as a means of gaining respite from the fighting, particularly if they were about to receive orders to advance. Prostitutes who were infected were able to earn high rates for passing on disease. There was no reliable cure for syphilis, but these men must have reckoned that a long-term risk was worth taking, compared with the odds of going over the top. When men were shooting themselves in the foot and swallowing septic matter in the hope of becoming ill enough to be sent home, then it is hardly surprising that such self-inflicted disease began to seem a viable option.

The sudden increase both in venereal disease and unwanted pregnancies meant that reliable forms of protection and birth control were needed, the latter term coined just before the outbreak of war by an American, Mrs Margaret Sanger.[24] In Britain a debate broke out as to who was responsible for the spread of infection, with young girls between 15 and 18 years of age more often blamed:

> The young women complained of are the product of our educational system
> ... Today hundreds of them are said to be little better than common prostitutes;
> but how can we justly attribute the entire blame to them? ... they have been
> ruined by men (many of them in the King's uniform) and no action has been
> taken against their destroyers. But the soldiers ... How can they be thought of
> as needing protection from girls younger than themselves? Who will ... restrain
> the polluters of our race?[25]

Crepe rubber condoms had been available since 1844, when Hancock and Goodyear had first developed the vulcanization of rubber process. Even after the quality of condoms had been improved,[26] making them more reliable, they were not disposable and so had to be kept clean, and washing and dusting them with antiseptic powder in wartime living conditions could be impracticable. There remained a great deal of ignorance and prejudice. A branch of the British Medical Association, for example, had passed a resolution in 1905 to make it an offence to advertise or sell and distribute literature concerning contraception. In France, a largely Catholic country, Jacques Bertillon formed the *Alliance Nationale Contre la Depopulation* (National Alliance Against Depopulation) to fight against the use of birth control as late as 1920, despite the experience of the war and the many children born out of wedlock.

In Germany, a Dr Richterhad had invented one of the first intrauterine devices, or IUDs, in 1909, but it had a tendency to cause infection and never caught on. There are accounts of German women during the war period, particularly in rural areas, drinking 'pot after pot of willow tea to prevent conception, or [they] drank it boiling hot to eliminate sexual desire'.[27] There were many folklore remedies thought to do the trick and in Britain raspberry leaf tea was recommended, both to avoid conception and, in sufficiently strong infusion, to bring about abortion.

In rural Europe, there was a tradition of cures being sold door to door by pedlars, but in Germany a rather euphemistic law was passed at the beginning of the century, to deter the traffic of condoms. Condoms, it was feared, might increase desire:

In conjugal intercourse the use of rubber articles could be intended for obscene purposes wherein pleasure is enhanced while the natural consequences are evaded.[28]

So, condoms were damned on both counts: for being contraceptive and for encouraging lewd relations. However, despite such laws for the general populace, the German army had been issued with condoms since the end of the nineteenth century. The Prussian army, despite the power of Catholicism, was keen to educate their mainly rural conscripts about preventative measures. Conscription concentrated the efforts of government on doing all they could to stop the spread of venereal disease, with the German War Ministry publishing information leaflets on condoms and salves, and organizing regular inspections in barracks. In due course, men returning home after the war were able to apply the methods they had learnt. In sum, the result was that 'the impact of the military as a social learning experience was most pervasive during wartime'.[29]

Britain, and later America, did not initially provide condoms to their troops, or promote their use.

For many facing the dangers of trench life, sex was a welcome release. The experience of war could be erotically exciting. Paul Fussell refers to Wilfred Owen's 'sensations of going over the top' as having an ambiguous sexual connotation, willingly exposing his body to enemy fire 'in the act of slowly walking forward, showing ourselves openly', as if, by implication, bullet and shell desire to make intimate contact with their victims.[30]

A German officer protests to his parents that his feelings of tenderness towards his men were not on any account to be interpreted as sexual:

I react very strongly to all external expressions; above all my worship of the beautiful is unbounded ... But I sharply separate my sexual and even my erotic feelings ... I have no feelings of love towards men, at any rate never sexual love, and I never shall have.[31]

When men were living at close quarters with other men, women with women, a sense of intimacy could easily grow up. In a war where a man's body could lie rotting and exposed in full view in no-man's-land, or where you could be chatting to someone one minute at a workbench and then she suddenly be killed by a defective shell – it is no wonder, in such an atmosphere, that old barriers against sexual expression might have seemed meaningless.

Earl Kitchener forthrightly advised every fighting man to be constantly on his guard against 'temptations both in wine and women. You must entirely resist both'.[32] When the American government saw the rise in venereal disease, it too attempted to promote abstinence, a tall order in the circumstances of war. An American military poster at the time declares:

> Only a poor boob pays his money, loses his watch, gets the syph, and brags that he's had a good time.

Risqué or pornographic pictures were popular in the trenches, but when objections were raised, whatever the official attitude might have been, little action was taken to ban them:

> Coquettish, flimsily clad ladies from French journals ... served as pin-ups ... Racier material was available from Egypt where an indignant missionary collected a sheaf of dirty postcards that were being sold to servicemen ... and [made a] demand for them to be banned.[33]

Brothels were well established in Belgium, and would adapt to serve changes in occupying armies, girls who had had the protection of a German officer, say, transferring to a British officer when the lines shifted, and vice versa. Reputedly German and Prussian customers were preferred by brothel keepers, in part because Allied troops earned less, so had less to pay for their services. A British soldier recalls that prostitutes would advertise by putting up notices on their

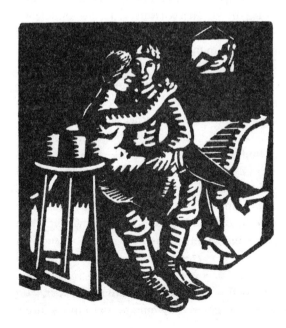

22. Sex in a Flemish brothel. Lino cut by William Kermode in Henry Williamson's *The Patriot's Progress*, 1930.

doors, 'Washing done here for soldiers'.[34] In France there are accounts of long queues, of hundreds of men, outside the legalized brothels, or *maisons tolérées*:

> I had seen a queue of 150 men waiting outside the door, each to have his short turn with one of the three women in the house … Each women served nearly a battalion of men every week for as long as she lasted. According to the assistant provost-marshal, three weeks was the usual limit, 'after that she retired on her earnings, pale but proud'.[35]

They provided not only sexual release, but also a welcome opportunity for men to socialize outside the parameters of military life. Some married men felt that they should discourage younger, inexperienced fellows from visiting prostitutes, whereas they themselves were merely keeping themselves shipshape for when they could return home to their families. Many young men, according to Robert Graves, preferred not to die a virgin. Married or not, clearly the experience was exotic for some of the men:

> There were about a dozen girls in there with hardly anything on and high heeled shoes. And they had little what they called chemises then. And they were sitting about on the troops' knees in all sorts of places. And apparently, the idea was that if you fancied any girl, you bought her a drink and then took her upstairs.[36]

Other accounts betray a sense of astonishment many felt at the contrast with both their previous experience of women and, often just a few miles from their trench billets, the elements of feminine luxury the women presented. Corporal Wood describes the 'seven young women … in the finest of flimsy silk dresses and then showing the daintiest of lingerie'. Private Eddie Bigwood is shocked to visit a house in Rouen where 'the ladies there had nothing on except a piece of lace … my eyes popped out'.

Brothels were segregated, with Blue Lamp establishments for officers and Red Lamps for the men. In some disputed areas officers from Central Powers and Allied forces might find themselves visiting the same places, but no officer would have thought it fit to visit a lower ranks' establishment or indeed vice versa. Neither would have felt at ease visiting the other's brothel.

Questions of Gender

A female munitions worker who had been presenting herself as a man, was exposed when she/he was called up. *The Times* newspaper found the fact that at the time she was going out with a young woman compounded 'the gender confusion by adding an issue of sexuality'.[37] While many chose to ignore the implicit questioning of set gender roles in cross-dressing, Willett Cunnington suggested that women dally with male clothing as a means of gaining status:

> He lends her his clothes to dress up in as he might lend a child his watch to play with ... [It is] when she claims them as her own that he disapproves ... for then such acts are immoral.[38]

Those women who chose to fight alongside men, including those who disguised their gender in order to do so, were more numerous than in any previous war. Though there are apocryphal accounts of men dressing as women to avoid conscription, perhaps it is unsurprising that it is cross-dressing women who had less reason to feel shame, at least in terms of cowardice, who were thus more likely to tell their story. To name but a few, Ecaterina Teodoroiu dressed and fought as a Romanian combatant, although, like Flora Sandes (see Chapter 3), she did not attempt to conceal her true gender; Wanda Gertz, by cutting off her hair and signing up in men's clothes, managed to join the Polish Legion on the Eastern Front as a man, under the pseudonym Kazik Zuchowicz; Dorothy Lawrence also managed to pose as a man in order to become a sapper, briefly clearing mines in the British Expeditionary Force, but she was only in the lines for ten days before she was discovered. Ironically she had signed up only in order to further a career as a reporter, yet after lengthy interrogation to check she was not a spy, she was allowed home to London on the understanding that she would not write about her experiences lest it threaten British security, the idea of women taking on male roles being seen as politically volatile.

The athlete Marie Marvingt is pictured in leather, fur-collared jacket and helmet, with long woollen skirt practically to the floor, as the first woman to fly combat missions as a bomber pilot. She is shown with skis in the Dolomites, serving with an Alpine regiment, and also, in a drawing by Émile Friant, attending to a wounded man with her proposed air ambulance. Her manner of dress is idiosyncratic but feminine, though early in the war she too had had to dress as a man in order to get to the frontline, serving with the 42nd Battalion of Foot Soldiers. Those women who succeeded in becoming combatants were acutely aware of the difficulty of negotiating a position where they could fight alongside men.

Women were thought to lack the killer-instinct, and it was feared that their presence would disrupt the ordered discipline of the ranks. If it was only in battle that man's true 'chivalry and sweet reasonableness [was] to be found',[39] how easily might their fighting spirit be displaced by any instinct to protect female soldiers, and thereby risk the majority? An added concern was that captured women might be raped and dishonoured. Conversely, the Russian authorities hoped that the presence of the female Battalion of Death would shame their increasingly reluctant male soldiers into more of a fighting, patriotic spirit.

Sexual Threat

A common fear in the German press concerned the behaviour of Allied colonial troops, lest their savage natures, their *viehischen Lüsten*, bestial lust, be let loose on blonde womanhood.

In prison camps older men and POWs were interned with women and children. These female prisoners and children suffered the same deprivations as the men, with dire hygiene conditions and next to no provision of clothing. A visiting Red Cross Committee in 1917 'did not approve of the presence of the interned women from Moravia on the grounds that these were an inevitable temptation for so many young, not all well-mannered or restrained men'.[40] To see the enemy as sexually voracious is a common fear in war, Christian Koller pointing out that similar sexual slurs were made by the Allied press:

> The way that the Germans portrayed the colonial troops was very like how the Germans were portrayed by the propaganda of the Entente powers.[41]

The French press, on the other hand, commonly infantilized their own Moroccan and Algerian troops, referring to them as *grands enfants*, or as over-sized children, perhaps because they were on the same side they merely belittled rather than vilified them.

Wounded Bodies

On the battlefields of the war, troops were not dying from a clean wound to the heart like the heroes in a comic book, but slowly from gas gangrene and trench fever, from typhus in the Balkans and septicaemia on inadequately provisioned hospital ships. Julia Kristeva drives home the point that coming face to face with our mortality in war is not a poetic metaphor signifying an abstract idea:

> A wound with blood and pus, or the sickly, acrid smell of sweat, of decay, does not *signify* death ... refuse and corpses *show me* what I permanently thrust aside in order to live.[42]

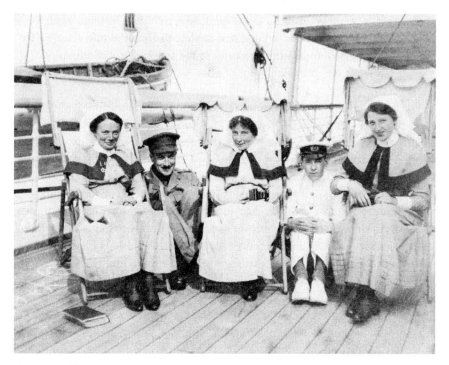

23. Nursing staff on HM Hospital Ship *Dongola*, in the Mediterranean during the Dardanelles campaign, 1915.

Antiseptics and mass inoculation against disease were possible for the first time.[43] However, antibiotics were not available until after the war, and in unhygienic conditions relatively minor ailments such as trench foot or surface wounds could develop, if left untended, into life-threatening conditions. When modern medicine was available, those who might once have died on the field of honour were returning home mutilated and shell-shocked. Those who died far from home might be left for weeks for all to see, in tortured repose on the barbed wire of no-man's-land, and as their bodies disintegrated their tattered clothing remained on their bones, helmets to mark the spot. The landscape has become the slaughtered men, 'Slashed and gouged and seared/Into crimson'.[44]

Even when still alive the bodies began to meld with the natural world. In a telling image a New Zealand artilleryman notices how a throbbing swarm of flies escapes from a dying man's mouth when he tries to exert himself. This was a common sight on the battlefield, known as the beehive phenomenon.[45] Again in apparent pastoral vein, a view towards the German line near Auchy appears to show a flock of sheep, grazing across the rough terrain, but they turn out to be:

Hundreds of khaki bodies lying where they had fallen in the September attack on the Hohenzollern [Redoubt] and now beyond the reach of friend and foe alike, and destined to remain there between the trenches till one side or the other advanced, which seemed likely for years.[46]

For those who did manage to return home, the ways in which they were received challenged any idea of unassailable male strength and independence. The beginnings of plastic surgery strove to help the severely maimed to regain a sense of autonomy. In Germany, the Prussian Jacques Joseph, working in the Charity Hospital in Berlin, performed thousands of surgeries attempting to restore facial features. The most common problems were shattered jaws, lost lips and noses and the gaping skull wounds caused by new weaponry. Joseph was one of the first surgeons to recognize the importance of aesthetic considerations for the patient. He wanted to question the morality that disfiguring wounds were something that had to be accepted, as a God-given trial, and that would be somehow unmanly to seek to put right.

In England, Harold Gillies, influenced by the work of the French surgeon Hippolyte Morestin, was keen to find the best methods of skin-graft surgery. However, his first major attempt at reconstruction on a British sailor in 1917 revealed just how aesthetically unsatisfactory early operations could be. Gillies himself treated over 2,000 men after the Battle of the Somme alone and his work influenced in turn the British plastic surgeon of the Second World War, Archibald McIndoe, who with the Guinea Pig Club gave hope to many severely burnt RAF aircrew.

When injuries were so devastating that no sufficient repair was possible, artists were employed to fashion prosthetic masks, so that these men might feel able to face the world again. It is a small irony that artists were also employed in both Central Powers and Entente forces to camouflage the new steel helmets and the 'beautiful military whiteness' of tents, creating a painterly illusion on and off the battlefield, but for very different reasons. Facemasks could be attached to spectacles, the frames holding them in place, to act as a visual distraction. A Ministry of Information photograph shows a patient of the surgeon Frances Derwent Wood at the 3rd General Hospital in Wandsworth, lost in contemplation of a plaster cast of his own face that is to be used to mask his injuries. The American sculptor Anne Coleman Ladd, working in a clinic in Paris funded by the Red Cross, made 'portrait masks' out of copper, which were then enamelled in skin tones to which human hair could be attached to disguise the telltale join.[47] The dental technician Archie Lane made similar painted masks at St Mary's Hospital in Sidcup, England, where over 5,000 servicemen had need of such help.

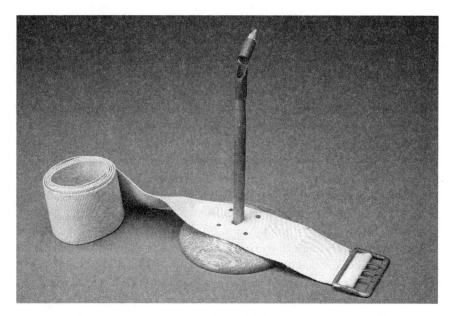

24. Prosthesis made for a man who had lost both arms at the shoulders, a rare injury even among the 41,000 British servicemen who lost one or more limbs during the war. When no limb stump remained there was no way of attaching an artificial limb. This simple device was strapped around the chest. The amputee would then write on a sheet of paper via movements of his torso. The device was invented by a Major Maclure, of the British Army.

Dental Concerns

Because so many facial injuries, particularly from bullet wounds, involved damage to the jawbone, the war also became a period of rapid advances in dental research. In America, for instance, Varaztad Kazanjian and Vilray Blair were experimenting with bone replacement surgeries. Such major injury apart, trench mouth, or acute ulcerative gingivitis, was a common complaint, involving painful gums and ulcers, leading to foul breath, crater-like cavities between the teeth and high fever. In the worst cases it could spread into the tissues of the face and the jawbone, resulting in deformities. The ailment developed in embattled conditions, with an absence of proper hygiene facilities, exacerbated by smoking and poor nutrition.

Such apparently small matters as an aching tooth could be overwhelming, even in the trenches. The poet Edmund Blunden talks of having to 'walk to Poperinghe in great misery to have a tooth put to rest or die in the attempt'.[48] A British NCO on the Somme in 1915 is more than prepared to resort to the basic dentistry available:

I broke a tooth while I was in the trenches ... The biscuits were very very hard ... I had a cracked tooth, a back tooth ... I'd cracked it on a rock cake two years before ... but in the lines it was agony ... Oh it got me! It couldn't have happened at a worse time ... I eventually found this man who was supposed to be 'the dentist'. I sat on a box ... a sergeant he held my head, put the half-nelson on me ... and an officer pulled my tooth with a pair of pliers. No water for rinsing. Instantaneous! I was really in pain, then, woof, all gone![49]

Despite what now seem primitive methods, the war brought many men dental care for the first time in their lives. Treatment may have been limited, but formed the beginning of dentistry for all:

We didn't have dentists in any great number in 1916. Then when the dentists came over and the men got their teeth put right, and the dead ones pulled out and so on, it certainly got them into another era of health, because their food could then be properly digested. It seems such a small thing, but it was of tremendous value when these dentists came ... Until then I don't think the public were as conscious of the value of teeth. And I believe it made a tremendous change in the attitude of the working classes after the war.[50]

A British POW in the Libyan desert feared that the dental treatment he received prior to the war might lead to trouble when he is recaptured by a group of Bedouins. A man's value was assessed in terms of clothing and whatever else might be harvested:

[They] soon went through my belongings and stripped me ... nothing of value, beyond my clothes ... though I was in some danger at one time by laughing and displaying my gold tooth. They appeared to think removing my head was the easiest way of getting it ... in the end I had nothing taken from me but a much-prized steel needle. I resisted by force, and then gave it to its would-be purloiner as a present. This made him very ashamed, and I hereby gained a friend.[51]

He manages to impress with the uniform he had hidden beneath his Arab disguise, and learns to entertain them by showing off his tattoos and that golden tooth. Another British officer manages to impress with a singular lack of teeth:

Civilized dental treatment always aroused great interest in this land of perfect teeth and I well remember an occasion when Lieutenant Tanner put the whole of our guards to flight by opening his mouth and letting his upper plate of false teeth suddenly fall.[52]

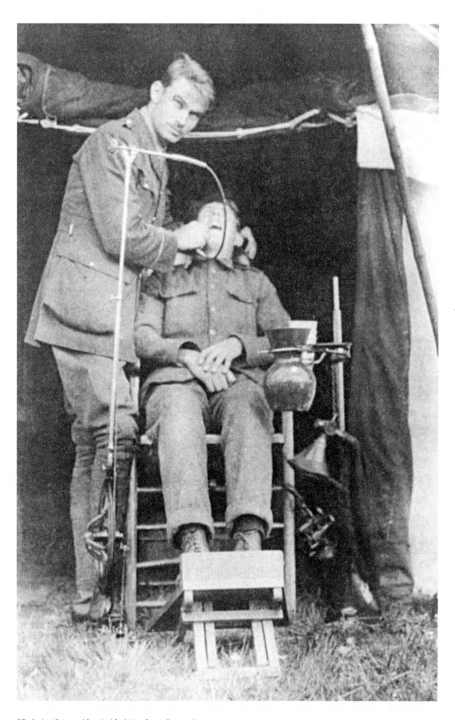

25. A dentist working behind the lines, Popperinge.

For those men who had entered the war with dental problems and those who lost their teeth in the war, more comfortable vulcanized rubber dentures became available, previously the preserve of the rich alone. The improvement and greater availability of dentures followed the path many relatively minor matters of appearance took, the war seeming to force the pace of discovery.

***

Given the devastating loss of limbs caused by the new more accurate explosives, there were advances in the manufacture of prosthetic limbs. Although wood remained the primary material used, lighter weight metal alloys were being developed. In Germany, at the Dresden *Einarmigenschule* (rehabilitation centre), Herman Perschel, who had lost both his right arm below the elbow and his entire left arm, is photographed playing cards and writing, wearing an artificial left arm that could be automated by moving his left shoulder; his right arm was fitted with a replacement hand. Jakob Veber,[53] of the Slovenian army, lost his leg while fighting on the Eastern Front in 1917, but continued to serve there until the end of the war. His wood, leather and iron-riveted prosthetic leg had two attachable feet, one for best and a stump for everyday.

Sabine Kienitz suggests that there was a marked difference in how the rehabilitation of male and female amputees was approached in Germany, with disabled women depicted in private at sewing machines or knitting, whereas men were shown in a public work context:

> The photos and texts suggest that the technical outfitting of the body and implantation of technology *into* the body was reserved for men only, because it was for them only that the enactment of labor and the staging of work ability was coupled with the technical enhancement of the body necessary to achieve it.[54]

In Britain, due to the thousands of men requiring limb replacement, the Queen Mary Convalescent Auxiliary Hospital at Roehampton came to specialize in orthopaedic cases, serving as a fitting centre. There were 200 beds by 1918. A Pathé newsreel at the time shows patients in their pyjama-like convalescent suits,[55] racing in wheelchairs and walking stiffly in a crocodile with artificial limbs and sticks, like some macabre conga dance. There follows a familiar scene of pretty nurses playing football with men on crutches. The men grin broadly at the camera, as if it is terrific fun to adapt to a new leg.

Unlike today, if you were unlucky enough to lose both legs, then there were no practicable prosthetic options. That said, given the range and

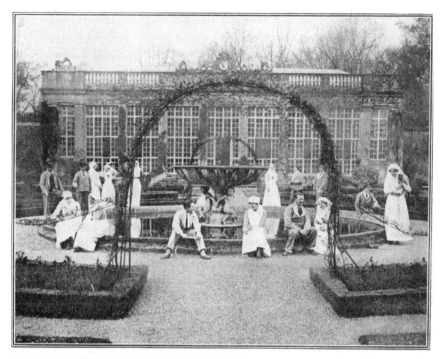

26. Convalescent British servicemen portrayed as if on holiday.

complexity of the injuries suffered, there were opportunities for customized invention. In the Wellcome Trust collection you can see, for example, a simple but ingenious device invented by Major Maclure of the British Army, for someone who has lost both arms at the shoulder, with no surviving limb stump to which a false limb could be attached. A canvas strap, which can be worn round the neck or trunk, is fitted with a pencil attached to a wooden disc, making it possible to write by movement of the torso, an idea which could be adapted for use with other tools (see Figure 24).

In America, anticipating the injuries that would ensue once they had joined the war, the Orthotic and Prosthetic Association had been set up in Washington DC in 1917. The wider use of the telephone meant that advertisements for prosthetic limbs were displayed in the new telephone directories, presenting a range of lighter weight and improved replacement limbs, even before the first American recruits had need of them. A case of pre-emptive strike advertising.

The Sporting Life

Both at home and on the battlefield there was a need for distraction – for sports, exercise and social events to motivate and keep people fit for the war. It might amount to rat catching with a terrier in the trenches, or learning to scud down the Euphrates in a native canoe. Despite all the hardships, for many, army fitness training and mess supplies meant being in better physical shape than ever before.

For women, the availability and social acceptability of more practical clothing meant that energetic sports could be taken up. British women working in munitions formed various sporting clubs, playing football, cricket, hockey, netball, tennis and taking part in gymnastics, running and swimming – activities that were unusual in most adult women's lives before the war. The first female football tournament was set up in 1916 in the north-east of England, 'popularly known as "The Munitionettes' Cup"'.[56] The AEC Munitions Factory team from Beckton, London, are pictured for their 1917– 18 season in masculine cotton jersey shirts bearing their logo, white shorts to the knee, thick socks, laced boots and a coloured mobcap with pompom, the goalkeeper in pale jersey and white cap. Significantly the knees appeared to be unhampered by stockings.

For cycling, women had worn bloomers or more often they had merely caught up their voluminous skirts. Now a farm girl working in men's breeches might ride a bicycle to work without hindrance. Swimming had been hampered by the restrictions of late nineteenth-century dress codes that had kept legs covered and bulky swimming skirts weighted with shot, to stop them floating upwards in the water. Catherine Horwood describes the popularity of swimming in pre-war Britain, though there was a reluctance to allow mixed bathing. There were random regulations as to dress, such as the insistence that all females over 14 should don an all-encompassing ankle-length robe or 'bath gown' for entering and leaving the water.[57] Women's bodies were thought more likely to arouse sexual feelings than 'exposure of the corresponding part of the male'.[58] Swimming costumes during the war became more streamlined than the layered frilly affairs of the turn of the century, particularly in fashionable seaside resorts such as Deauville and Biarritz. Yet, even there, female swimmers were still wearing fairly cumbersome frocks to the knee, worn with bloomers and often with two pairs of stockings beneath, topped with a helmet-shaped hat.[59] Jersey fabric, developed in America, allowed swimsuits much greater freedom of movement, but was not widely available until after the war.

At the Wimbledon tennis tournament in London, women players were provided with a rail in their locker room on which to hang their blood-soaked steel corsets.[60] Unlike other female tennis players of the period, Suzanne Lenglen left off her corsets, to give herself greater ease of movement. Though her career was interrupted by the war, she played her first French Championships in 1914 at the age of only 14, and was already demonstrating the sartorial flair that was to make her a totem of sophistication in the early 1920s.

Football provided a short period of respite for German and Allied troops on Christmas day 1914. As the British troops climbed out of their trenches in response to the German invitation to suspend hostilities, their officers warned them that it might be a trap. They went all the same, and 'we shared goodies with the Germans and then from somewhere a football appeared'. They knocked a ball about together, one soldier recalling that 'it wasn't a team game'.[61] Just outside Ypres, it had not been a time for taking sides.

Football could be a means of rallying the troops, as when Captain Willy Nevill of the East Surreys, hoping to encourage his men to go over the top, suggested they kick a football between them all the way over to the German defences. The ploy succeeded, and the two balls used were brought back to England as mementos, though Nevill himself had been shot and killed.

***

For all its devastating consequences, despite those permanently disfigured or psychologically damaged, war brought for many a fitter body and opportunities for new social and sexual experience.

6 ENTERTAINING COSTUME

In Paris, Berlin and London the need for entertainment was answered by numerous variety and cabaret shows. Designers would press the most beautiful stage entertainers to wear their clothes. Even if you could not afford to get to the theatre their images on advertising billboards and in newspapers and magazines influenced ideas of the ideal fashion look of the moment. In the trenches, for example, cigarette packets contained cards, or in the case of German cigarettes the packaging itself bore such images. Series such as Gallagher's *The Great War* (1915) depicted scenes of the war including images of the trenches, barbed wire and shrapnel hitting a wall, which could be collected and exchanged and then sent home to feed a child's collection, perhaps. Wills' *Musical Celebrities* (1914) or sets of *Beauties* connected to a world distinct from the theatre of war, of familiar actors, film stars and models. In the first months of the war Allied cigarette cards were printed on silk with a paper backing, but due to shortages of materials, by 1917 production ground to a complete halt and they were replaced by paper cards.

The actor Gladys Cooper became the most popular pin-up for British troops and sales of her picture postcards were particularly sought after. Prior to the war she was shown in rich materials, with pearls and fox furs, whereas her wartime clothing is more often demure, wishing Happy Birthday in a soft-collared white day blouse and plain tailored jacket say, and in many she is shown with her daughter, as the good and dutiful mother. In one, both woman and child are wearing sou'wester hats and voluminous raincoats, for seamen far from home, perhaps.

***

Cabaret in Germany during the First World War was heavily censored, the authorities at first uncertain whether or not it should be allowed to take place at all during the conflict, which they assumed would be short-lived. When the war became protracted cabaret was reinstated, driven by the need to keep up morale, and importantly here, it relied on its association with luxurious, carefree dress:

> To the extent that it was contemporary, topical, and *aktuell*, cabaret dealt primarily with fashion, with current styles and trends.[1]

In Berlin cabaret and theatre was determinedly light-hearted. Costumes were intended to provide glamour and escapism, in stirring 'inflammatory orgies of nationalism'.[2] Light operas and musicals were popular fare with Fritzi Massary, an Austrian actor and singer, renowned for her 'talent for clothes' as the journalist Elsa Herzog opined.[3] With many struggling to survive high inflation, and malnutrition rife on the streets of Berlin, figures like *die Massary* (the Massary) as she was known, with her highly feminine ensembles of lace and silk, feathers and jewels, provided an image of the glamorous lifestyle that one day might be attainable by all.

On the other hand, in the theatre women were often portrayed as stay-at-home figures, rather than sophisticated fashion mannequins. The writer Friede Kraze's 1915 *Erfüllungen* (Fulfilments) was a drama played out within the confines of a German home, and typical of the way in which women were presented when 'scenes of quiet domesticity dominate over scenes of battle and political activity'.[4] Unlike cabaret, here the women were soberly dressed, in long dark skirts with corseted high-buttoned bodices, practical low-heeled boots and hair severely scraped back into neat buns.

Munich's café culture provided a measure of social commentary, with highly stylized artists such as Marya Delvard. Her extravagantly vampish appearance, with sleek body-hugging costumes, often in black against a startling white face, caused the writer Hans Carossa to remark that one could not help but think 'involuntarily of sin'. From 1912 she appeared in the *Simplicissimus* cabaret, where the atmosphere was satirical and to some degree critical of the prevailing nationalism. Delvard and her husband Marc Henry would sing duets dressed as French revolutionary peasants, he in nankeen trousers and cap playing a guitar, she in a full cotton chintz frock, bloomers and poke bonnet, referencing perhaps German rural life and the possibility of dissent among the working classes.

In London the big musical hits of the war period seem curiously exuberant, and irrelevant. *Chu Chin Chow*[5] was a lavish affair based on the tale of 'Ali Baba and the Forty Thieves' in *The Arabian Nights*, involving Eastern-influenced costumes, with men in gorgeously embroidered side-toggled jackets and black satin breeches, oriental caps and long thin moustaches; women in a variety of billowing, gilded and embroidered silk trousers, tiny bustiers and splendid plumed headdresses embellished with veils, bells and snakes, straight out of the wildly influential Ballets Russes *Scheherazade*. In contrast the cast of the revue *The Bing Boys are Here*,[6] starring George Robey and Violet Loraine, was largely in contemporary dress, the two 'boys' of the title kitted out like matching Charlie Chaplins, in too-short trousers, too-small pudding-basin hats and childish round-collared shirts, suggesting both innocence and empty pockets. Their audience was swelled by working women now able to afford to go out in their new finery, in ersatz silk blouses and boaters done up with long black velvet streamers and poesies all round, bent on enjoying a night out at the theatre. Sometimes they might be accompanied by men on leave, in uniform perhaps to avoid being 'feathered', who might well have enjoyed the chance of a little showbiz gloss, rather than anything more critically demanding.

Artists like Vesta Tilley found the war provided them with new opportunities, with stirring shows where she would encourage young men onto the stage to sign up, gaining for her the sobriquet of 'Britain's Best Recruiting Sergeant'. Tilley was renowned for her *en travesti*, or drag king roles, often playing a toff, in white tie and tails with a tipped-back top hat, singing 'Burlington Bertie' perhaps, an aristocratic young ninny. On stage, even when playing foolish young men, she is said to have carefully maintained an aura of femininity; off stage she was dressed in gorgeous gowns, furs and expensive jewellery. As the war progressed she took to dressing as uniformed Tommy in the Trenches or Jack Tar Home from Sea and performed in hospitals and convalescent homes. In both guises, in mocking the upper classes or as a cheeky Tommy who knows how to look after himself, she allied herself with the majority of the wounded – and the mass of working men who fuelled the war effort.

American vaudeville followed a similar pattern of seemingly carefree entertainment, heavily sponsored by links to the fashion trade. Manhattan cabarets had been forced to close at two in the morning in 1913, encouraging the growth of private clubs that could get round such restrictions. The dancers Vernon and Irene Castle, who had an enormous influence on the birth of the dance hall, set up their *Sans-Souci* Paris-style venue in Manhattan's Times Square in 1915, but unlike more traditional family-orientated vaudeville, this was entertainment for adults only, serving the 'fantasies and desires of adult men and women'.[7]

Yet the popular image of the Castles was one of respectability. Irene Castle lent her name to numerous advertising campaigns, from cosmetics to cigars. When the couple popularized ragtime music, making dancing up close and personal seem acceptable behaviour, then her image of smart shingled hair, or what became known as the Castle Bob, and shorter length skirts, became respectable too. Her fancy for seed pearl necklaces also became fashionable

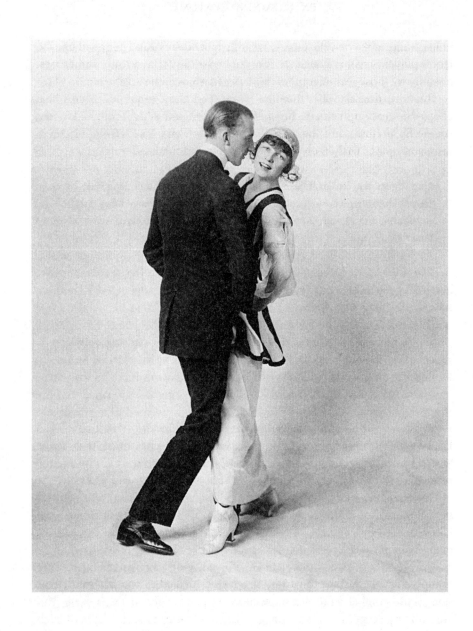

27. Irene and Vernon Castle dancing up close, c.1913.

in her wake, and when she took to wearing a bandeau round her head like the tennis player Suzanne Langen, it was dubbed a *Castle* Band – and sometimes, possibly by those less tolerant of the flux of fashion, a headache band.

Ragtime dances were the new craze and they required clothes that allowed for easy movement. Before the war the Castles had brought African-American rhythms and the Argentine tango to Paris. In Philadelphia there were attempts to cash in on tango fever, advertisements offering

> 'tango shirts' and 'tango shoes' for men and 'tango sashes' and 'tango hats' and even flexible 'tango corsets' for women. Bolts of brilliant orange fabric that had sat around in dry goods stores flew off the shelves when the color was dubbed 'tango'.[8]

The artist Sonia Delaunay created her own take on a tango outfit in 1913, her artist husband Robert Delaunay also taking up the challenge. For her first such dress she wore

> the *robe simultanée*, a gown made of pink, scarlet, blue and orange sections, which she wore to dance the tango with her husband at the fashionable Bal Bullier. Robert wore a red coat with a blue collar, a green jacket, a sky-blue waistcoat, a red tie, red socks and black and yellow shoes.[9]

In London too tango caught on. Christmas 1913 saw exhibitions at the Prince's Hotel and Ballroom, one clergyman muttering sourly that it was 'one of those animal dances that have no *raison d'être* but to gratify animal passions'.[10] Tango was even banned by the Pope. It became wildly fashionable in Germany, the Kaiser ordering his army and navy to refrain from dancing both the tango and the two-step, because of the lewd behaviour and dress it encouraged in women – or risk dismissal. Had he been taken seriously, it might have proved a pleasant means of avoiding conscription.

In Paris, home of the cabaret, links between the fast-growing haute couture fashion business and the theatre were well established. Uniforms from either side of the conflict were not allowed on stage, or indeed the depiction of any military scene, for it was thought that the 'desire to forget is obvious in the theatre and it is as much the result of government propaganda as of the public's eagerness to be entertained'.[11] However, the presence of the war and the geographic proximity of the Western Front meant that it could never have been far from people's minds. A growing awareness of the squalor and loss of life was in mute ironic contrast to the fanciful costumes and light-hearted manner on stage.

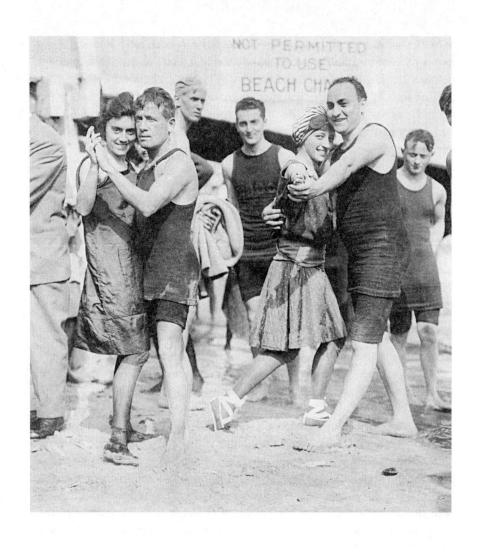

28. The tango was all the rage on Brighton Beach, Brooklyn, New York City.

Theatre Companies in the Field

In 1917, there were 25 English-speaking acting companies alone performing scenes from Shakespeare, Sheridan and Shaw in France, touring behind the lines.[12] With many theatres closing in London after the outbreak of war, some women did venture into the lines to entertain the troops. Gladys Cooper – doyenne of the cigarette card, and already a well-known face, along with the actor-manager Seymour Hicks – took a small company into France, dubbed *The National Theatre at the Front.*

Female entertainers in particular were there to raise morale, but also to act as a reminder of the mothers, wives and girlfriends they had left behind, and the standards of gentlemanly behaviour required of them. When the American singer Elsie Janis performed in France, in hospitals, from the back of trucks or from table tops, she wore primly fashionable suits with perhaps the addition of a Doughboy helmet for a touch of added sauce. The perceived danger was that in consequence of forming a fighting force, an absence of personal accountability might make men, anonymous through uniform, forget how to behave towards a woman.

Concert parties of conscripted men adopted costume and make-up to perform when the conflict allowed. The Jocks of the 15th Division, for example, performed in dark Pierrot suits,[13] white ruffs and skull caps, whereas the Balmorals of the 51st Division Entertainers[14] are pictured dressed in baggy clown costumes with pompoms down the front and powdered white wigs. One of their number is shown being dressed by a local French woman, her long dark modest dress contrasting with the performer's frilly pantomime frock, long ringlets and heavy stage make-up.

Both Entente and Central Powers within POW or internment camps often took part in ad hoc productions to pass the time, in costumes adapted from whatever fabrics and accessories that could be attained. At the 360 POW Camp in France, three German prisoners are shown in tall pointed hats and all-in-one clown suits made from painted sacking, worn with pompoms sewn onto slippers and army boots.[15]

The presence of clown figures in so many of these companies was a traditional element of variety troops. As wise fools or fools who inadvertently speak the truth, with their pasted on sad expressions and crocodile tears and their guise of physical powerlessness, they might well have seemed like a commentary on their circumstances, whether as POWs or as troops waiting in the lines.

On the home front, small-scale amateur shows were organized to entertain wounded troops. The suffragette movement,[16] for both strategic and patriotic reasons, adapted their pre-war suffrage pageants to support the

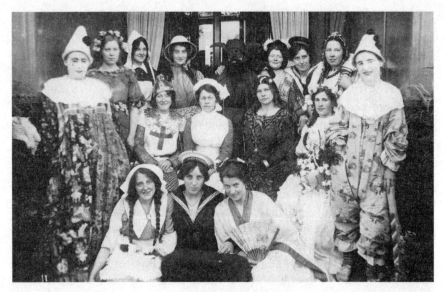

29. Nurses got up to entertain patients in a cabaret, with dressing gowns for kimonos and knitting needles through their hair, their red crosses acting as the cross of St George with knitted armour and clowns in borrowed curtains.

war effort. Convalescent homes organized fancy dress parties, often involving impromptu cabaret, a long way from the sort of high society party where costumes were prepared far in advance. Photographs of wartime hospital entertainments show nurses in Pierrot costumes fashioned from curtains, dressed as soldiers or sailor boys in uniforms probably borrowed from the men they were nursing, or got up as geishas in dressing gowns with knitting needles through their hair. George and the Dragon could be achieved with the witty addition of a helmet and the suggestion of chain mail via a crocheted bolero, thereby reinterpreting the red cross on the front of an apron. Their young faces are lined up and smiling alongside the bandaged men with pinned up trouser legs and empty jacket arms.

***

The relationship between the Ballets Russes and haute couture relied on the extraordinary visual impact of the costume designs of Léon Bakst and, to a lesser extent, Alexander Benois. Previously ballet had involved tutus and pink satin pointe shoes, with male dancers kept in the background playing primarily, and literally, a supporting role, to hoist the ballerinas on high. Suddenly men were centre stage, in gorgeous often erotically suggestive

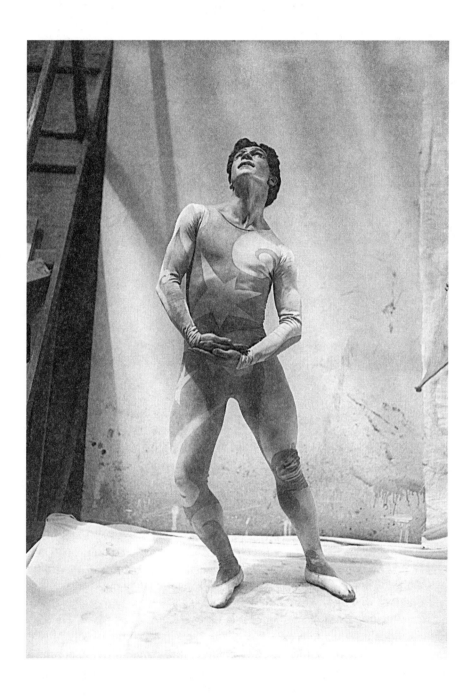

30. Male dancers centre stage, in the Ballets Russes production *Parade*, Paris, 1917.

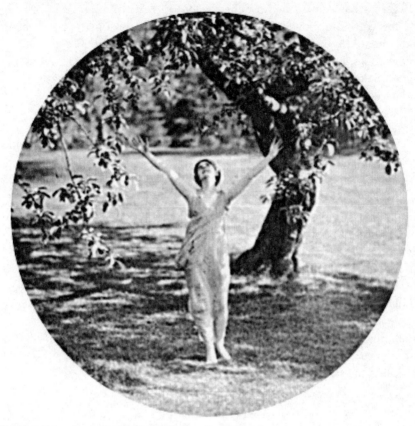

31. Isadora Duncan dancing in a simple Grecian toga, at one with nature.

clothing that appeared to reveal bare flesh, even when this was in fact merely the illusion of flesh-coloured cloth, quick changes often making this a practical necessity.

However, on occasion it could be the Ballets Russes who were astounded by their audience, rather than vice versa. During their successful run in pre-war London, Diaghilev was puzzled by a strange sound, a 'barely discernible noise' emanating from the audience that he could not at first place. Then he realized what it was: 'the public was gently clapping its kid-gloved hands'.[17] Despite their delight in the jewelled colours and exotic designs, a British audience of the affluent classes was apparently unprepared in 1911 to express itself more demonstratively. However, within a week the Knightsbridge department store Harvey Nichols 'cleared their windows of the white, cream and lilac of summer fashion and filled them instead with hangings in Bakst purple and red'.[18]

Isadora Duncan opened a dance school in Paris in 1914. Although the war forced her to move back to America, the impact of her appearance in performance, in uncorseted fluid white togas and with bare feet rather than pointe shoes, not only influenced dance but also can be seen in the tiered demi-toilette evening dresses at the beginning of the war, with necks left unfettered by jewellery as if mimicking Greek statuary.

The interplay between fashion and ballet worked in both directions, with fashion designers like Paul Poiret and later Coco Chanel designing for ballet and theatre, and Bakst, working principally for the ballet, designing clothes for the couturier Jeanne Pacquin. Pacquin in turn went on to help modify costumes that at the last minute proved to be impractical for Nijinsky's ballet *Jeux*.[19] The artist Natalia Goncharova, who designed fabrics and decorations for the Ballets Russes incorporating her elaborate ornamental appliqués, was employed post-war by Marie Cuttoli's avant-garde fashion shop, Maison Myrbor. A design concept for costumes for a ballet, such as Sonia Delaunay's for Diaghilev's production of *Cléopâtre* in 1918, could then be marketed to the fashion world, promoting 'Egyptian' style dresses. Delaunay opened a boutique in Madrid in 1919 selling pared down versions of her designs, simple shapes appliquéd with geometric and circular forms in her signature brilliantly contrasting colours. This two-way collaboration between ballet and fashion brought greater fluidity and perhaps dramatic impact to fashionable dress, and the skills of the atelier to ballet design.

***

Turning to the illustrations of much fashion and ballet design, Georges Lepape's renderings of Poiret designs[20] focus on elegance of silhouette, and their colour palette is rich but often subdued: a bruised murky purple gown, a deep grey-green coat with huge black fur collar, all set against a striped wallpaper of the same grey-green and turquoise; a dark blood-red shift with a geometric pattern at bodice and hem worn with a deep purple turban, the figure standing to one side as if to make way for a blank almost two-dimensional white room. The wide collars, sweeping capes and helmeted haircuts seem stark in their landscape, as if despite the beauty of line and colour it apes something of a gaunt wartime world.

In *La Gazette du Bon Ton*, a drawing of Poiret's 'La Robe Blanche' by J. L. Boussingault in 1914 is in contrast a slight black-on-white line drawing, of a plain tunic-shaped elongated bodice and four-tiered crimped skirt. One hand rises to her neck and the small masculine hat is set at a becoming angle. In all these sketches the female body beneath the clothes is hardly discernible, apparently an afterthought. While haute couture is at the forefront of what seem to be clothes allowing corset-less fluidity, the reality of the body beneath is withheld.

In the case of Erté's figures, however, the body becomes a more substantial presence and often the flesh is coloured in. Even when all we see is a finger pointing from a Magyar (batwing) sleeve, we are made aware of the bust and hips present beneath.

Anne Hollander describes designs that allowed for more fluid movement as evidence that 'for the first time in history the look of comfort and freedom became elegant'. This change is greater than its material parts, the 'liberating violence of the shift in fashion almost inconceivable to the modern world, [was] like the corresponding shock which attended the First World War itself'.[21]

In the years before the outbreak of war, Paris haute couture was becoming established worldwide, through designers such as Lucile (Lady Duff Gordon). Her pretty gowns were given emotionally charged names, such as 'The Sighing Sound of Lips Unsatisfied' or 'Red Mouth of a Venomous Flower'.[22] Lucile had a flair for business. With opportunities limited in Paris because of the war, she concentrated her attentions on her American boutiques, regularly showing her designs on Pathé and Gaumont newsreels. By 1916 she licensed a fashion line in the Sears Roebuck mail order catalogue, selling at way below her usual couture prices. She also wrote a fashion page and columns for Hearst newspapers in both *Harper's Bazar* and *Good Housekeeping*. The latter helped her reach out to a less affluent – and potentially larger – market. She was the first to hold mannequin parades, creating a social occasion to show off her newest designs. Ahead of her time in packaging too, she designed boxes smartly striped in green and white, and customized with her signature.

Madeleine Vionnet is said to be responsible for bias cut skirts, which allowed women to wear figure-hugging clothes in which they were still able to move. Hollander suggests that it is only since the First World War that 'women who do nothing at all have been officially despised'.[23] New fashions may have allowed greater freedom of movement, but they were usually depicted suggesting a leisurely lifestyle and thus in line with a more traditional aristocratic manner of dress. In this context, while vampish female actors may seem more up-to-date in that they were more obviously sexualized, the prim-looking clothes of Mary Pickford seem more suitable for a job of work, and therefore do not suggest a leisured class.

However, it was Chanel who was the outstanding innovator of her age. Fundamental to the idea of haute couture was that designs should be one-offs, requiring enormously wealthy customers. Chanel turned this idea on its head, designing simple elegant shapes that were easy to copy: in *Vogue*'s terms, producing Ford-signed Chanels. Mass-produced clothing techniques had of necessity become more efficient and streamlined during the war, due to the need for uniform. Chanel's designs lent themselves to the assembly line. Everyone with an interest in fashion could buy themselves a little black dress, yet somehow the most desirable, the most likely to transform you was a *Chanel* little black dress.[24]

Chanel used sports-influenced jersey fabrics, derived from Jersey fishermen's wear, which had been considered unsuitable for haute couture because it was difficult to sew and ornament. Poiret, on the back foot, said of her that 'her women resemble little undernourished telephone clerks'.[25] Chanel accepted that it was the war that established her, claiming that 'in 1919 I woke up famous'.

Unlike male couturiers, Chanel – by virtue of gender free from the draft – was able to stay open throughout the war, her shop in Deauville, opened in 1913, becoming a watering hole for the wealthy, specializing in women's sportswear. By 1915 she was doing well enough to open another boutique in Biarritz, drawing in the custom of those who had moved there to escape the conflict, close enough to an escape route into neutral territory should the progress of the war threaten their safety. *Vogue* magazine describes a life of indulgence, oblivious of what was going on at the fronts:

> One dances, swims, plays tennis and goes to the Casino in the evening; there are races in September and a horse show in the winter, and there is fox hunting in the fall.[26]

By 1916, Chanel had extended her reach across the Atlantic, and become hot news in the American fashion press. Ironically perhaps, it was this surge of American money that gained her entry to full couturier status in Paris, the magazine *Les Elégances* publishing a swathe of her separates in 1917, her shorter skirts and blouson belted jackets 'emerging as the hallmarks of her everyday style'. Mary Davis locates Chanel's success both in her embrace of everyday fabrics and her empathy with new movements in art – towards a focus on architectural line and interest in the underlying structure of a garment, over surface decoration.

Men not in uniform might purchase a new lounge-tuxedo suit, available off the peg, to wear to a nightclub. Chanel's take on suits for women in turn influenced more comfortable 'lingerie' soft-collared shirt styles for men. The ubiquity of the simple skirt suit for women, sometimes with waistcoat, was itself influenced by the variety cheeky-chappy female performers. Moreover the simple boxy cut, often with loose dropped waist and self-fabric belt, had much the look of the men's new service uniform designs. The growing popularity of these softly tailored suits goes to explain British *Vogue*'s autumn edition in 1916, which featured VAD and FANY uniforms, practical uniform become desirable high fashion.

Despite the isolation imposed on America from the beginning of the war, due to the difficulties of supply lines to and from Europe, the influence of Parisian designers still held sway in the domestic market.

The Influence of the Silver Screen

If clothes need to be seen in motion, on the body rather than in graceful impressionist sketches, then film newsreels on the streets of the main combatant cities at the time come into their own. They reveal women with skirts rarely much short of the ankle and men, when in civvies, uniformly soberly dressed. Designers working in the fashion industry, as much as those from theatre and ballet, were quick to see the commercial advantages of working in the film industry. The silver screen brought larger than life images of desirable clothes to a far wider range of possible audience, though the direct effect on ordinary fashion could be hard to decipher. It was more often evident in the sudden popularity of small accessories that the impact of a film star say, would make herself felt. A ribbon half undone at the neck, a way of tousling your hair might seem to turn you into Lillian Gish, or a pastel washed silk chiffon scarf could take on for a moment the elusive quality of a Fortuny-dressed siren in exquisite pleated Delphos sheath. These illusions are at the heart of fashion.

In the new medium of film, actors such as Gish and the enormously popular Mary Pickford favoured an *ingénue* appeal with their long ringlets and wide-eyed innocent expression. When their skirts were short, it was more to do with playing very young, rather than suggesting more emancipated practical dress. At the birth of Hollywood's influence on fashion, with cinema fast becoming the entertainment of the masses, their sensitive, somewhat pert, faces on sandwich boards and hoardings promoted an image that was childlike and largely conservative in manner and dress.

Theda Bara's image, on the other hand, was more worldly. While Gish and Pickford sport Peter Pan collars, sometimes frilled *Papillons* (butterfly) frocks and neat feminine suits with often a glimpse of petticoat, Bara earned her nickname of The Vamp. Her image in *Cleopatra* is mature and sultry, with kohl-rimmed eyes and for its day, shockingly revealing exotic clothing, drawing attention to breast and crotch. In a publicity photograph of 1917 there is nothing coy about her appearance: her face is shown close up and intense, her gaze distracted, suggesting a complex inner life, a raven winding itself about her neck and staring at a woman who pays it no attention. She posed as the Serpent of the Nile with live snakes and skulls, and with long, pointed fingernails.[27]

Far from an image of romance or of mother figure, the influence of Ballets Russes designs was again evident. It is not the civilizing femininities of dainty lace trimmings, but fur and feathers that frame her, suggesting savage nature. This was the first sex symbol female film actor, and what she wore, or did not wear, encouraged a generation to want to ape her languorous appeal. The image combines motifs from the past with contemporary fashion, the exotic with the cute, as when she wears an Egyptian-style pharaoh headdress with little-girl ringlets, a dress with fairy-like wings and embroidered flowers over each naked breast and crotch. This deliberate ahistorical abandon is reminiscent of contemporary designers like John Galliano, who draws on a vast range of theatrical and historical sources in apparently wild juxtaposition.

In contrast, the enormous popularity of cowboy films in the silent film era – or Westerns, a term coined in 1912 – might be said to herald the beginning of European fashion's enthusiasm for casual clothing, particularly for men. Riveted jeans, trouser belts, open-necked shirts, pull-on boots and casually tied bandanas were the forerunners of what now seem fashion staples. There is something too in the cowboy's nonchalance, gently blowing down the barrel of his gun or correcting the angle of his Stetson before riding off into the Wild West, that carries forward to the laid-back sophistication of tough guy Hollywood stars like Humphrey Bogart, with his withheld snarling grace, as he tips his fedora and leaves the room.

Yet the stronger contrast here is with the First World War, for the cowboy was also a cipher for the soldier, world weary, dressed in clothing that had endured a long ride across treacherous terrain and in the face of evil gunslingers out to kill. The image of the cowboy ennobled them and made them not one of an army but individuals every one.

7 MANUFACTURE AND THE HOME

W ar produced a need for fabric for the body of aircrafts (see Chapter 4), for tents and groundsheets, and for sheets and bandages for the wounded. Most of all vast quantities of cloth were required for clothing, for military uniforms and for new civilian and quasi-military roles. But then war went and disrupted the delicate balance of pre-war trading agreements, making fabric increasingly hard to come by. Fortunes were made in the scramble for wool and cotton from fresh sources. Before the war there had been long-established arrangements between the now combatant countries. Britain had provided good quality wool and robust leather for shoes and boots, with Bulgaria, say, reciprocating with its silk and cotton production. Germany produced fine leather for shoe uppers and brought its new expertise to artificially engineered fibres and diverse haberdashery items. In 1914 all khaki dye used for British Army uniforms was imported from Germany. Russia, for example, had difficulties ordering British cloth when it was fighting on the Eastern Front and supply lines had broken down.

When khaki dye was obtainable, there could be difficulties working with the cloth, as a machinist found working at Schneiders in London. At first she was trained up to use the new industrial machines on paper instead of cloth, before being trusted to sew khaki. The work was hard and the chemicals used in the dyeing process give her 'khaki poisoning', a form of blood poisoning:

> What with being undernourished ... I suppose everything built up ... I had boils, one under the arm, one on my back. Dreadful one on my arm like an apple ... The Doctor said he'd have to lance it and when I came back it had burst ... Time off work? If you stopped to blow your nose you got the sack![1]

As Germany had industrialized later, it had the advantage of benefitting from Britain's example; its machinery and technological methods were thus more up to date. By the 1900s Germany had replaced natural or vegetable dyes with those derived from coal tar. The major German chemical cartels before the war, known as the Big Six, predecessors of the vast I. G. Farbenindustrie conglomerate founded in 1925, provided most of the world's supply of synthetic dyes. Indeed it has been argued that the dye and chemical industry was a major underlying cause of both the First and Second World Wars.[2]

A by-product of dye production happened to be TNT, and because of its military potential, huge stockpiles had been built up for the production of ammunition should a war ensue. This fuelled confidence that Germany was in a position to win. Moreover, America was almost wholly dependent on Germany for its supplies of pharmaceuticals, dyes and other chemical products. When America joined the Allies in 1917, this provided an opportunity to break free from Germany's monopoly and to begin to develop its own chemicals industry.

However, in 1914, America was still importing up to 90 per cent of its requirements, and was anxious as a neutral nation to secure its supply lines. For instance, in the first months of the war, Frank Woolworth made a request to the British First Lord of the Admiralty, Winston Churchill, for permission to use spare storage capacity in Atlantic convoys, to carry luxury goods from Europe for America, including those from Germany to America. He was given short shrift, Churchill arguing that British ships laden with American goods would be less able to evade German U-boat attack. Finally those already purchased were loaded and safely delivered to America and Woolworth's Five-and-Ten (dollar) stores, but no further passage was made available.[3]

For domestic use in Germany, *Papiergewebe*, or paper cloth (mentioned in Chapter 4) was produced as a cotton substitute used for underwear, such as *Leibchen* long stocking supporters, which resembled a vest with taped ties, worn by boys and girls until adolescence. The paper textile was even used to make soft toys, and although it is hard to find evidence of its durability or otherwise as clothing, as substitute boot soles it proved of little use for troops on long marches or in wet conditions. Production certainly fell off after the war.

The German submarine *Deutschland* was launched in 1916, unarmed and with, for that time, substantial storage holds, in an attempt to break the Allied blockade. On its first outing it carried amongst its cargo 125 tons of dye components and drugs, including the recently developed treatment for syphilis, Salvarsan – all bound for Baltimore. However, after a number of American freight ships were sunk by U-boats, trade relations broke down with Germany. Eventually the *Deutschland*, along with a number of other merchant U-boats, were converted for active service in the German navy.

A by-product of the German chemical dye industry was chlorine gas, used as a weapon in trench warfare. Phosgene gas proved more lethal, and eventually it was combined with chlorine, though mustard gas was

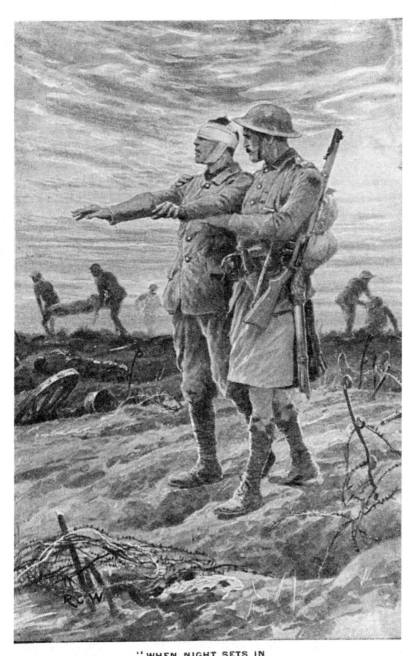

"WHEN NIGHT SETS IN
THE SUN IS DOWN."

From the painting by R. Caton Woodville.

32. Postcard of one soldier leading another, blinded and bandaged, through the battlefield. On the back of the card, masseur is suggested as a suitable profession for blinded soldiers from the front.

discovered to be most effective. It was less easy to detect and had the practical advantage of remaining active in the ground, effectively clearing areas for weeks. Despite protestations from Sir John French, the British Chief of Staff until the end of 1915, who blamed the Germans for playing 'a very dirty "low down" game', the Allies were in fact quick to follow suit and use chemical warfare. The injuries and manner of death could be terrible, with loss of sight and excruciatingly painful burns. There were sometimes delayed effects, with victims becoming 'yellow-faced and choking'[4] and eventually suffocating. However, it was not only the symptoms but also the idea of an unseen, vaporous weapon that could not be fought against, that spread terror – even though from a statistical point of view it was relatively insignificant. Gas attack caused only 5.7 per cent of non-fatal injuries and 1.32 per cent of battle deaths during the course of the war.[5]

The need for protection led to a series of gas helmets being hurriedly developed. Before these were available

troops were instructed to dampen any available piece of material – a handkerchief, a sock, a flannel body-belt – and tie it across the mouth and nose until the gas passed over.[6]

After a chlorine gas attack, men had to improvise as best they could to alleviate the symptoms, recalling the John Singer Sargent painting, *Gassed*, 1919, which records the aftermath of mustard gas:

Our eyes were streaming with water and pain, and all we had was a roll of bandages in the first aid kit we carried in our tunic. So we bandaged each other's eyes, and anyone who could see would lead a line of half a dozen or so men, each with his hand on the shoulder of the man in front.[7]

The British Hypo helmet had a loose flannel skirt soaked in anti-gas chemicals, which unfortunately had a tendency to drain away in rain, and a celluloid window, which could steam up, making vision difficult. Robert Graves finds it of little use:

A greasy, grey felt bag with a talc window to look through, and no mouthpiece … the talc was always cracking, and visible leaks showed at the stitches joining it to the helmet.[8]

The box respirator was more effective, and many versions were tried out, such as the Russian *Zelinski*. The German army initially wore goggles and cotton gauze pads soaked in bicarbonate of soda, urine or plain water.

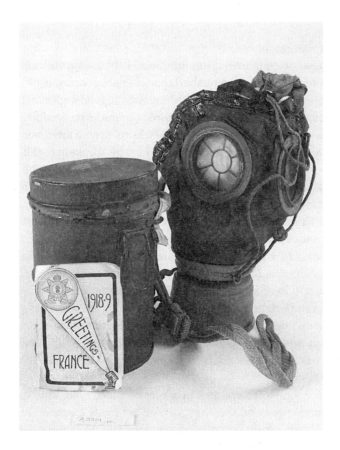

33. German canister gas mask with container and Christmas card, 1918.

Piete Kuhr describes new gas masks in 1915, carried by the soldiers passing through her German town, close to the Russian front:

ugly, snout-shaped, grey-green masks with glass windows to see through and a supply of oxygen for breathing. When a poison gas alarm is raised at the Front the soldiers immediately snatch their masks from their belts and cover their faces with them. But the warning often comes too late.[9]

In Britain the *Daily Mail* newspaper ran a campaign to get readers to make pads for Allied troops. By 1916 *The Great War* magazine claimed that all British packs carried 'smoke and tube' helmets. The new helmet, 'the goggle-eyed booger with a tit'[10] had a valve held in the mouth and better protection for the face at least. In America a filter was developed made from peach stone and walnut shell charcoal, and a nationwide campaign in 1918 got women and children collecting and sending in both stones and shells.[11]

***

As soon as America began to prepare to join the war in 1917, the production of uniforms and other textile goods meant shortages of quality materials for domestic consumption. The mills in the South and in New England undertook to supply the war effort, and exports of raw materials to the main body of Europe were therefore curtailed. However, large stocks of luxury fabrics in Paris meant that well-to-do civilians were still catered for by the ateliers that remained open.

Attempts were made by Central Powers to continue trading with America since they were suffering shortages of basic materials for their war effort. Once it became clear that the war would not be over quickly, they were in desperate need for saltpetre for gunpowder for example, and cotton for clothing and even bandages for the wounded. Cotton had come mainly from India, Egypt and from America, but all these sources had been cut off by the British naval blockade, and in this respect the Allies were better off.

Although there were shortages, there was no formal, across-the-board clothes rationing in any of the participant countries during the First World War. Advertising campaigns sought to raise awareness of the need to limit civilian textile usage, and manufacturers were encouraged to conserve resources for the war effort.

The new machines designed for uniform production, which were able to prepare cloth with greater speed and accuracy, cutting out many garments at the same time, derived from recent paper production processes. This meant that the role of the traditional tailor or skilled seamstress came under threat. Relatively unskilled women workers could be taught to man such machines. Moreover the fashion for more simply shaped clothing, with loose-fitting A-line shirt dresses, say, that therefore did not need to fit exactly to the individual figure, lent themselves to mass-production. A shorter, narrower skirt used less cloth.

Shopping

Women's fashions were influenced by the restrictions imposed, yet more practical clothing for both sexes, or clothing that at least had the appearance of greater practicality, was already beginning to be fashionable well before the war. It follows that this tendency cannot be explained, or at least not entirely, by the war. Economic conditions and a sense of moral Puritanism towards sumptuous dress at such a time are contributory factors, though luxury goods continued to be desired and bought and worn. *Punch* magazine

ECONOMY IN DRESS: THE NEW SMARTNESS.

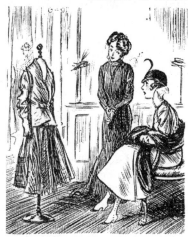

"It's lovely, but I'm afraid thirty guineas is too much for me."

"It is a good deal, but Madam must remember this is a genuine old dress. We guarantee it to have been in constant wear for at least five years."

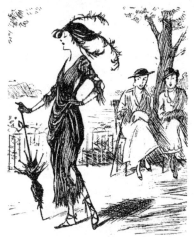

"I say! that's a smart frock, if you like!"

"H'm, yes. But it's only imitation—not real old."

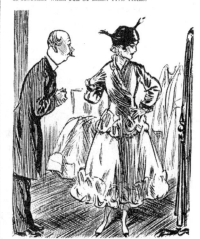

"I like it, but it looks dreadfully new."

"If you feel that, Madam, might I suggest that you have it soiled by our special process? We only charge three guineas extra."

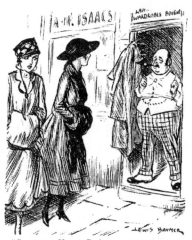

"Come along, Mabel. Don't make your mouth water looking in there. Old clothes are not for the likes of us."

34. The desire for a patriotic well-worn style. *Punch* magazine, 12 April 1916.

has two elegantly dressed women intimidated by another in plain uniform-type suit and hat in March 1916,[12] and by April, in a series of cartoons by the same artist, women are yearning for the most worn-out, second-hand-looking garb. A woman in tatters is observed by two others:

'I say! That's a smart frock, if you like!'
'H'm, yes. But it's only imitation – not real old.'[13]

The Great War magazine in July 1916 links this attitude with a response to having been at war for two long years:

It became bad form to be garish or sprightly in costume. To wear old clothes was regarded as a sign of patriotism.[14]

Imagine the cities of Europe and their new large department stores, where you might browse for goods. In England and Germany, such shops had at first been designed for the upper middle classes, and it would have felt uncomfortable for those of evidently insufficient spending power to enter such exclusive establishments. War meant women from the working and lower middle classes suddenly had spending power, though in Germany, where women were not initially mobilized for war work, this was less the case.

Department stores like Selfridges in London encouraged this new market. Even women with less disposable income could glimpse what money could buy. They could see for themselves – touch or even try on clothes that they might one day realistically aspire to own. A lower middle-class woman working as a secretary might reasonably hope to afford a Jeanne Pacquin-style evening dress, or a working-class woman budget for a fur coat out of her munitions wage, with no husband at home to question her decision. With plate glass windows to display the goods, window-shopping became a popular pastime, the art of the window dresser to entice passing trade. However, in wartime Britain this was no longer possible at night – when clothes can seem at their most tempting – as window lighting was prohibited. Harry Selfridge's attitude to selling embraced the modern idea of customers delighting in shopping for its own sake:

I want them to enjoy the warmth and light, the colours and styles, the feel of fine fabrics. That is the basis of [my] business.[15]

Although American-born Selfridge's offer to assist the war effort was not taken up by the British, the French government awarded him a contract to supply all their army with underwear, and he gained respect by refusing commission on the deal. He was an advocate of advertising continuing throughout the war:

> War requires two forces: one of men who fight, another to carry on the work of making and providing. The order of the day must also be advertising as usual.[16]

The consequence of this policy meant that he was to make vast profits throughout the war period, and mostly, as far as clothing was concerned, from less expensive lines.

It was already common before the war for copies to be made of Parisian designs. Poiret, for example, set up the *Syndicat de Défence de la Haute Couture Française*, the French Haute Couture Defence Union, to limit this practice. In Germany there were similar attempts to thwart piracy, through organizations such as the *Verband zur Förderung der deutschen Hutmode*, the Association of Förderung German Hatters. Germany had ambitions to rival the domination of Paris and London, and there was a call for a national German museum of clothes and accessories, led by the architect and decorative arts shop owner, Ernst Friedmann, in the spring of 1915.[17]

Poiret saw the commercial potential of selling licences for his designs to be reproduced under his label, thereby maintaining some control over what was sold in his name. However, as with today's 'knock-offs', more often they would be counterfeit enterprises, of poor quality, with the charismatic name doing the selling rather than any genuine connection with a designer's skill.

In America, American designers were producing their own work for the new and thriving ready-to-wear market, but often selling under a French label. Given the embargos on foreign trade, and with Paris taken up with the business of war, previous arrangements were thrown into confusion. In the period from 1914 until preparations began for America to join the war in 1917, when home grown textile supplies were still readily available, there was a chance for these American designers to come forward under their own names and circumvent Paris. There was a concerted effort from the fashion press to encourage home grown talent, and competitions were held to find new designers to take over the reins. The editor of *Vogue,* Edna Woolman Chase, arranged a fashion show in New York to promote American design, christening it a 'Fashion Fête', as if the name would help achieve a sense of style comparable to the French. Leading retailers like Henri Bendel were invited to produce collections, to be shown over three days, for the benefit of Allied widows and orphans. Journalists set out to appeal to the public's and the manufacturers' sense of patriotism, but it was 30 years before the idea was taken up, after another world war. Paul Nystrom remarks that American design failed to grasp this pivotal opportunity:

> At the very time when it might have attained a greater importance, due to the isolation of France from the rest of the world by war, the movement itself had been deemed hopeless by American producers and distributors.[18]

Ideas from Paris continued to hold sway despite the war:

> By the start of 1915, American fashion advertising and retail catalogues reflected how quickly the United States ready-to-wear makers had responded to the stylistic changes introduced by the French just a few months earlier.[19]

For those who lived far from the city in America, mail order catalogues such as Sears Roebuck and Montgomery Ward had been a lifeline from the latter years of the nineteenth century, providing patterns of designs from Europe, as well as ready-to-wear garments. A version of a wedding gown designed by Chanel in the spring in Paris could appear in a catalogue in America in the summer, and be worn by a bride in rural Kentucky by early autumn, and at a fraction of the cost. If there was no money to spare, then the array of illustrations were fashion education and entertainment in themselves. Even before the 'roaring' twenties, Sears had begun to market its clothes using film stars to endorse them in full-page advertisements. Men are sometimes depicted wearing Western-style Stetsons and boots, borrowing the aura of the fictional cool cowboy figure that cinema had established as an iconic image (as detailed in the previous chapter) even for those city-based Americans whose lives had nothing to do with the Wild West.

Advertising was a cost effective means of inducing demand, using not only billboards and print but also radio, the latter becoming much more popular during the war, partly in order to keep in touch with the war's progress. When America joined the conflict in 1917, all commercial and private radio use was banned. War imposed restrictions on advertising, as too obviously promoting luxurious lifestyles could seem in poor taste against the backdrop of loss of human life. An advert in 1918 for the Chicago firm of Chas A Stevens and Bros, for example, has models for sportswear, an intrinsically leisure/luxury idea, in two-piece suits that mimic military uniform in their severity, detail and dark colours. The narrower skirts and shorter hemlines, however, seem excitingly new, under a headline stressing their practicality:

Utility Sport Suits
SMART – SIMPLE – DURABLE[20]

***

This was the dawning of the age of electricity, and better lighting meant that clothes could be made more easily at home in the evenings, causing less strain to the eyes. While modernized clothing factories might have the benefit of electric lighting, sweatshops that continued to make up short runs and supplement seasonal fashions were sometimes not so fortunate. Moreover, young women, or rather young eyes, were a requirement of the dressmaking trade, since lighting was often kept deliberately low in order not to damage the cloth. When much clothing was black, which is particularly difficult to sew without causing eye strain, the situation became worse. Arthur Marwick suggests that the war was a disaster for the 'sweated' dressmaking trades, although some of these women were able to find work in armaments and other factories during the war at least.[21] The majority of piecework, often carried out by working-class women who were either tied to the home or could not find full-time employment, remained as it had long been, poorly paid work in dire conditions with no security.

Women not otherwise involved in the war effort were encouraged to sew and knit for the troops, rather than dress hats or tat cushions, providing in the main socks, underwear, sweaters, scarves and blankets, fostering a sense of solidarity and helping them feel practically useful. Charitable sewing and knitting was in part an indicator of means. Claridge's Hotel in Mayfair London, for example, held sewing circles to make uniforms and clothes for the poor,[22] the Red Cross providing kits for making 'hospital garments', advertised as 'cut out free of charge',[23] a hobby activity for the better off.

Just as sewing machines had transformed pre-war fashion production, now they were able to meet the need for uniform for the services. The division of labour in a garment's make, breaking down its manufacture into a number of small, circumscribed tasks,[24] saved time and therefore expense, but also meant there was less need for experienced hands. For example, in a mass-production line of service tunics, one person might cut the pattern out, another sew the main seams, another make and fit collars, cuffs, epaulettes and pockets, another make the buttonholes and finally yet another sew on the buttons. If this series of processes was further broken down, the make became even more efficient. Increasingly specialist tailors were going out of business, leaving only those catering for the small moneyed minority who could still afford hand-tailored coats and suits, and for the ultra rich who could still buy couture.

Thrift had become a patriotic duty. Women's magazines and dress pattern companies promoted the idea of mending and adapting old clothes. *Neva*, a pre-revolutionary Russian magazine along the lines of the American *Ladies Home Journal*, issued multi-printed patterns with pattern pieces for several garments, one on top of the other and graded for size, which could then be traced, perhaps onto newspaper.[25] In Britain in 1918, with supplies running low, a much simpler template was produced for a National Standard Dress, which met with little enthusiasm:

> A 'utility frock' with a vengeance, built economically without hooks or eyes or metal buckles, the one pattern designed to serve indifferently as 'outdoor, housegown, rest gown, teagown, dinner gown, evening dress and nightgown'. It does not appear to have secured the popularity such a portmanteau-garment deserved.[26]

The pattern pieces were designed to fit neatly together, minimizing waste of both fabric and paper.

Men's civilian suits had jackets slightly shortened, sleeves and trouser legs narrowed and unnecessary detailing such as pleating removed. For the proficient dressmaker, double-breasted coats and jackets were adapted and cut down to single. The skirts of pre-war dresses could yield enough fabric for a simple smock dress, though often what had been considered suitable stuff for a day dress now lent itself more easily to evening wear.

Knitting and Sewing for the Front

Homemade comforts, and in particular warm, comfortable clothing, could make all the difference to men living in wretched combat conditions. In Schneidemühl, a war savings collection is spent on wool: 'We must now knit woollen things for the soldiers'.[27] In Doubs in France, schoolteachers produced over 4,000 hand-knitted balaclava helmets for the bitter winter of 1915.[28] Knitting took over from embroidery as a lady's pastime. It could confirm your patriotism, proving you no longer saw yourself as someone at leisure. Campaigns were launched in Britain and later in America to encourage women to knit for the war effort, and patterns were issued in newspapers and women's magazines. The Women's Legion, for instance, knitted socks and jumpers for Lady French's Fund for soldiers overseas.

Knitting was a traditional homely pastime, often undertaken by the elderly and infirm. Propaganda film coverage now showed young working women knitting socks for the war in their lunch breaks, and wounded male

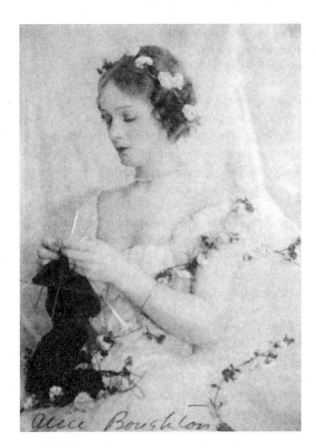

35. The dancer Adeline Genée, on tour in America in 1914, found knitting socks for soldiers in the wings between acts.

convalescents being taught to knit by their nurses. The Red Cross published patterns suitable for the front, warning that knitters had to adhere to their guidelines or the clothing would not be suitable, and even able-bodied men in non-combatant roles were pictured with knitting needles akimbo. In Philadelphia a poem captured the mood, where knitting is a way of dealing with the anxiety for those engaged in fighting, 'In train or tram [I] knit and knit/Sometimes the newsboys hurry by/And then my needles seem to fly'.[29]

In Australia, where knitting circles were particularly well organized, a spiral sock pattern was developed, its lack of fashioned heel meaning it could be knitted more easily. Moreover, it lasted longer because the point of wear was not always in the same place.[30] American children joined knitting clubs, the least proficient still able to take pride in producing squares for surgical wipes. The double-knitting process enabled more able knitters to knit two garments at once,[31] even the complexities of conventional socks negotiated on the same set of needles. The American Fund for the French Wounded together with the Red Cross put out an appeal for warm shawls for the thousands of French women made destitute by the war.

Knitwear, which had formerly been worn by children in the main, was now warm clothing for land workers and the military. This in turn led to civilians adopting jumpers and knitted accessories. Cunnington remarks on the craze for hand knitting, mentioning the 1917 fashion for women's jumper blouses, which could be slipped on over the head without fastenings, 'and the jumper coat, hip length, with loose fastenings' and the variant 'jumper frock'.[32] Fair Isle, sleeveless pullovers for younger men had begun to be worn even before the war, and the intricacy of the ancient patterning and its individually performed stitches, which required considerable knitting skill, lent itself to the idea of gifts of symbolic worth for men at war. Colourful jumpers worn underneath a service tunic were both warm, and also a way of making that uniform feel more individual to the wearer.

Even in the trenches men had to darn their worn out woollen socks, cobble together ripped uniforms and re-stitch buttons. A batman would take on this task for his officer. The Salvation Army and Red Cross stations attempted to provide the material and emotional comforts of home, from cakes and tea, 'the art of the winsome, attractive coquetries of the round, brown doughnut and all its kindred',[33] to such 'womanly' activities as washing and mending their clothes. To have someone prepared to take on such small intimate tasks was in itself a reassuring kindness in the harsh situation of the trenches.

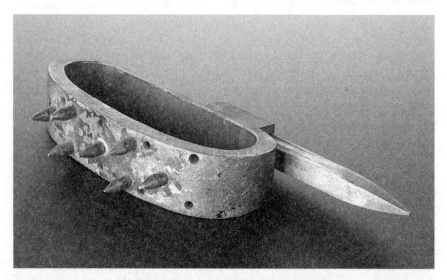

36. Many took unofficial weapons into the field. This knuckle-duster would have been worn for man-to-man combat, perhaps carried on night raids. The retractable blade measures 60mm.

The Great War magazine lauds women of all classes for sewing and knitting for British soldiers in the field:

> Every woman in the land, from the Queen down to the humblest labourer, was engaged in some sort of needlework guild to provide shirts for soldiers, socks for the men in the trenches, mufflers for the sailors keeping watch on the North Sea. There was scarcely a thing likely to be needed for the fighting men that was not made by the million by the women of Britain.[34]

The apparent cosiness of these sewing and knitting circles could not belie the underlying tragedy of war. A generation of young men were being killed, and the women who might well have taken pride in their new communal enterprises were aware of this truth. A poem evokes an older woman who has lost her son, and now knits for others:

> I'll shape the toe and turn the heel
> And vary ribs and plains
> And hope some soldier-man may feel
> The warmer for my pains.[35]

***

Children from all sides played their part in providing for the war. A French poster proclaimed:

> Children are emptying their woollen stockings, breaking into their piggy banks, counting their pennies [for] clothes to save [soldiers] from the cold. Dressings for the wounded.[36]

A German poster shows a small girl cutting off her doll's hair for a Red Cross collection, to make felt for lining military helmets.[37]

Children helped prepare parcels for the front, sewed and knitted for the soldiers, wound bandages, helped with clothing collections, folded and packed laundry for the Red Cross, and cut out dressings from cotton waste, organized through their schools, or often scout and guide organizations. Since Robert Baden-Powell's influential *Scouting for Boys* published in 1908, the scouting movement had spread to British territories and also to America, Northern Europe, France, Germany and Russia by 1910. The focus on militaristic uniformed discipline and practical outdoor activities lent itself to the war effort.

The scout movement had uniforms remarkably similar to the new army service uniforms, with loose blouson top, neckerchief, felt campaign hat, sturdy boots, and with epaulettes and insignia that had a distinctly military appearance. Indeed, in America, Congress agreed to make a special case of their scout uniform, when it was changed from navy blue to khaki in 1914, having otherwise banned civilian uniforms that resembled the army's.

Children at Home at War

The war could all too easily provide the imaginative basis for children's game play. A. J. Halliday's *War Games for Boy Scouts*, published in 1910, caused many to volunteer when war broke out. Winston Churchill, First Lord of the Admiralty, was of the opinion that war should be approached as an extension of school games. Boys reared on ideas of the honour and excitement of fighting for one's country were eager to volunteer before the war might be over, the National Service League claiming that, in Britain alone, 15 per cent of those recruited were in fact underage. For most children war-themed games and toys were a natural response to the conflict. Toys could be a problem though, with a schoolgirl in England advised by her grandmother that sacrifices would have to be made, taking away 'all our toys that were made in Germany, amongst them a camel, of which I was very fond'.[38] Even children were required to take sides.

There was a surge in sales of toy soldiers, dressed in replica uniforms. The National Doll League Children's Unconscious Doll Exerciser was advertised in the *Daily Mail* in 1915. The boy's version consisted of a soldier doll with sprung arms and khaki uniform, trousers, jacket and cap, and was said to provide health-giving exercise to the child. Girls could have one kitted out as small boys or as nurses, as it was considered gender-appropriate for them to play at mothers or nurses, though it is curious that it was considered inappropriate for girls to have had a soldier doll to tend. Jennie Lee, future British politician and 10 years old when the war broke out, relates how she and her friends thought up a 'fascinating new game' using their broken limbless dolls to represent wounded soldiers.[39] Piete Kuhr is more of a tomboy, playing soldiers with her friends so frequently that their mothers complained of the damage they were doing to their clothes. Piete's solution is to 'only wear my gym knickers or a discarded pair of shorts from Willie's [her brother's] sailor suit. This is much more convenient'.[40] A British girl is given a toy nurse by a soldier leaving for war, but finds she cannot bring herself to play with it, and puts it instead on the mantelpiece, in a position of honour.[41]

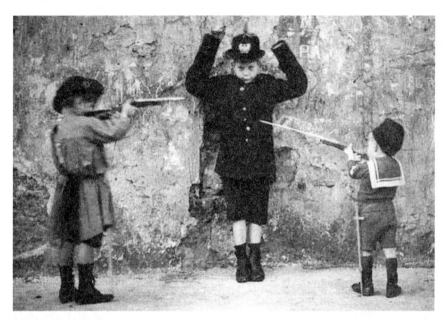

37. Children dressed for war.

Often dolls were intended as propaganda items rather than for children to play with, as with 'Convalescent Blues' or 'Hospital' dolls, made for the British retail chemist *Boots* in 1916, sold to raise money for war charities.[42] On all sides patriotic toys were produced for children. In Britain toy tanks were on the shelf only six months after they were first used in battle, 'in France, Lusitania jigsaws and a militarized version of Monopoly; in Germany miniature artillery pieces which fired peas'.[43] Paper cut-out dolls were perhaps the least expensive toys marketed. A child could dress them up in any of the various belligerent uniforms, and as actual uniforms changed or different nations come to the fore, then they could easily be exchanged.

POWs on both sides produced toys, carved dolls and articulated models from scraps of wood, to send home to their families or to raise a little money for the small items that made camp life more bearable. Possibly an outlet for the frustrations of captivity, some of these toys seem unsuitable for children, such as a German tank carved from chalk by an Italian POW at Flexecourt camp in France in 1919[44] or a wooden model of a kilted soldier towing a POW by the neck with hands tied behind his back.[45]

There are many images of children in the war period dressed in miniature versions of adult uniform, and these may in part account for the attraction, for some children, of joining the scout movement. For the children of the upper classes, fancy dress parties were the rage in London:

> But this year [1915] the frivolous columbines and harlequins, the troops of elves and fairies so popular in peacetime, had been ousted by fleets of juvenile sailors, contingents of small red-capped nurses, battalions of miniature soldiers shouldering toy rifles – even a six-year-old Admiral, wearing a small cocked hat and sporting a little sword.[46]

For the less well-to-do, scaled-down children's field service uniforms were available 'for as little as 5 shillings and 11 pence'[47] from the London store Gamages. In the fractured terrain of Belgium and Northern France children may not have been in the position to enjoy toys and costumes bought for them, but they could still pick up discarded pieces of uniform and adapt them for their games.

Children's activities, their toys, games and what they wore, were all affected by the war. One English schoolgirl, just six in 1914, and living near a hospital, remembered seeing 'soldiers in their blue uniforms and red ties – such a lot of them it seemed to me'.[48] A Viennese woman for whom the cost of war was high – one son dead, one blinded and another who had lost his reason – two years after the end of hostilities comes upon her grandchildren, whom she thanked God would be spared the travails of her sons' generation, and what are they about? In soldiers' caps fashioned from newspapers, playing at war all over again.[49]

8 DEATH, MARRIAGE AND IDENTITY

Clothing could be a means of expressing grief, providing some comfort for the bereaved and signalling what might be difficult to express in words.

Black Mourning

In the nineteenth century the rules of mourning dress had become minutely circumscribed, where income allowed. In Britain the influence of Queen Victoria's 40 years of mourning had seeped into ordinary bourgeois clothing values so that black was a respectably safe choice across the board. The details of appropriate mourning dress were laid down concerning each and every family relationship, and at what precise period of time after death they should be changed, from, say, Paramatta wool tweed cloth, to crepe, to silk and crepe, in minute gradations to half-mourning and finally back to ordinary dress. Children's mourning clothes were also black and often deliberately restrictive, made of fine fabric to honour the dead, suggesting that a bereaved child would have no desire to play.

In the First World War black clothing was thus at first adopted for civilian mourning dress, and with black armbands worn over uniform. There are accounts of the streets of Paris, Berlin and London abruptly turning black. Lady Duff Gordon, of the couture house Lucile, notes this sudden transformation:

> In one week Paris was a changed city. The streets were full of women dressed in black; the churches were crowded all day long.[1]

In provincial Germany, Piete Kuhr remarks that one Sunday in 1914 the church in her town 'was full of people wearing black clothes and black mourning veils'.[2]

France, in part because of its long Catholic tradition, and significantly here including fashionable France, remained loyal to the traditions of mourning, continuing to wear black until as late as the Second World War. The editor of American *Vogue*, Edna Woolman Chase, describes its countrywide imposition:

> In a country where heavy mourning had long been a tradition [it] seeped like a dark tide through the towns and countryside as the casualty lists came back from the trenches and funerals were the macabre social life of the capital.[3]

Mourning clothes for women were intended to demonstrate a retreat from sexual feelings and express a need for seclusion, though the latter at least was impossible for women who needed to work. The nineteenth-century widow might eventually remarry, but it was held as important that after the death of her husband she appear as if a new emotional life was far from her thoughts. However, in the First World War efforts to demonstrate lasting respect for each individual began to have less meaning in the context of such mass bereavement.

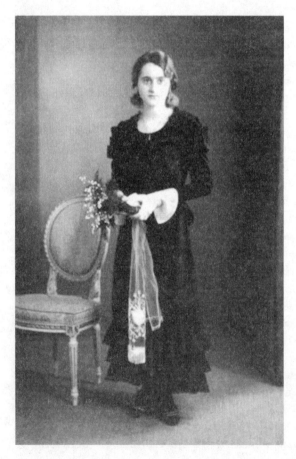

38. Courtauld crepe tiered mourning dress, worn with white lace veil and silk gauntlets, a bunch of lily of the valley, known as Mary's tears – as in the tears of the Virgin Mary at the crucifixion of Christ.

Thus, as the war progressed and the losses mounted, mourning dress began to be less widely worn. Relentless black mourning could lower morale, both for soldiers coming home on leave and for the general public. Moreover, severe fabric shortages meant that it could be prohibitively expensive to acquire a new dark wardrobe, and even to dye what clothing you had was beyond the means of many. There were attempts at alternative ways of expressing loss, such as wearing purple armbands and *The Times* correspondent in Germany reporting a plan to substitute black dress mourning with a scarf pin, as a more discreet token.[4] The older generation continued to wear black both in and out of mourning. They were usually less in the market for new clothes and if they were, they tended to be more conservative in their choices. However, black was becoming more widely worn for elegance, for ordinary office daywear and even to express the erotic. It began to seem less associated with mourning and its absence therefore no longer necessarily betrayed a lack of respect.

Despite this gradual shift in attitude, the British firm of Courtauld's, who had built a worldwide business manufacturing mourning crepe throughout the nineteenth century, continued to supply Britain and much of Europe throughout the war. When death could come at any moment, all manner of fabrics and accoutrements such as gloves and mourning hats, with black, lilac and grey silk flowers still manufactured in France, needed to be readily available.

Increasingly the ready-to-wear market, with the more standardized simple shift-style dresses, meant that mourning could be bought off the peg. Courtauld's made vast profits through the course of the war, taking out costly full-page advertisements and employing fashionable designers, such as Lucile, to display their fabric in *Les Modes* magazine.

A fashion advice column in the French magazine *Femina*,[5] which ran throughout the war, suggested that dress had become more truly chic and more streamlined through the deprivations of war. Mourning, it claimed, need not fall short on style when you might sport the shorter skirt, albeit in black with, say, a becoming little hat made from black ribbon worn with long gloves ornamented with chains made from copper wire. The apparent understatement and discretion of mourning dress could play on the age-old attraction of what is covered up drawing all the more attention to the wearer, and those aspects of a person that are apparently withheld. A chic mourning veil would encourage the onlooker to wonder about the face that lay beneath. This is not necessarily to suggest cynical or trivial reasons for adopting black, but rather that interest in the power and nuance of fashion choices played their part, and were perhaps a welcome distraction at times, even if the bereaved adopted mourning.

Out of mourning black emerged Chanel's plain black simply cut dresses. Roger Boutet de Monvel's cartoon in the *Gazette du Bon Ton*[6] shows six stages of a French widow's mourning, from *Grand Deuil* (the deepest stage of mourning), in elegant little clean-lined tunic dress, heavily veiled and hiding her face behind a black handkerchief,[7] then a white handkerchief, gradually bringing herself to powder her nose, apply lipstick and finally to wear a pale dress with fur cuffs and beaded black trim, cigarette in hand – aptly demonstrating the ability of haute couture to take on mourning. Lou Taylor enumerates the first stage of fabric worn as wool and crepe with veil, the second *Petit Deuil* as allowing black silk taffeta with dull-stoned jewellery and finally ordinary mourning with black crepe and pearls or diamonds.[8] Chanel's 'Little Black Dress' (as discussed in Chapters 6 and 7), in black crepe with long slim sleeves, was to become the new uniform of seduction and bereavement, a dress for all occasions in fact, that could be replicated in factory mass-production copies across the cities of the West.

Mementos

As for what might resurrect the memory of individual soldiers or nurses for those at home, medals and official letters of condolence might on occasion have been less affecting than a comb still clogged with hair, a worn toothbrush, or a length of webbing scrubbed smooth with Khaki-Blanco by their hand. If a kit were returned home after someone's death, such items as these might well have taken on a poignancy beyond their apparent value.

Vera Brittain was well aware of this practice, for it had been the subject of letters in the papers; but upon receiving the kit of her fiancé Roland Leighton, the reality of his death is expressed through the simple eloquence of uniform and small personal possessions, telling the intimate story of life in the trenches:

> There were his clothes – the clothes in which he came home from the front last time – another set rather less worn, and underclothing & accessories of various descriptions. Everything was damp & worn & simply caked with mud. All the sepulchres and catacombs of Rome could not make me realize mortality & decay & corruption as vividly as did the smell of those clothes.[9]

The small extravagances Leighton had carried to France are evidence of his need to maintain his old self in the chaos and carnage. It was his own body heat that had managed to protect what felt most important, even when all else had been invaded by corruption:

All that was left of his toilet luxuries came back – a regular chemist's shop – scented soap, solidified Eau-de-Cologne etc. We no longer wondered why he wanted them. One wants the most expensive things money can buy to combat that corruption. Even all the little things had the same faint smell, and were damp and mouldy. The only things untouched by damp or mud or mould were my photographs, kept carefully in an envelope, & his leather cigarette case, with a few cigarettes, a tiny photo of his mother & George Meredith, & the three little snapshots ... of us, inside. He must have had those things always on him, & the warmth of his body overruled the general damp.[10]

White Mourning

By the end of the war so many had been killed that white was sometimes adopted rather than black as a symbol of mourning. In the last phase of the Roger Boutet cartoon white is worn as if it were colour alone that had to be avoided.

The wearing of white to express grief might be looked upon as an echo of the deepest mourning of medieval European queens, or recall perhaps the simple white chemise dress worn by Marie Antoinette at her execution. When Emily Wilding Davison was buried, her suffragette friends wore white, often associated with purity and innocence as opposed to the sophistication of black, together with black armbands and carrying bunches of white arum lilies. Black risked seeming too hackneyed for a new cause; white suggested a desire for a new order of response that might be less conventional, and more keenly felt. Yet white had long been worn in many non-Western countries as traditional mourning dress, and there were even examples in Europe of white being worn for funerals.

The custom of the Death Wedding remained, where young people who had died were buried in white, as if to suggest the virgin bride or groom going to her or his spiritual marriage, in death. It was the custom in France to bury young women in white with orange blossom wreaths and in southern Germany they were buried in tall crowns, sometimes initialled 'J' for *Jungfrau*, or virgin.[11]

Marriage and Weddings

With so much death, marriage was the counter-balance. It could express a belief in the future. A wedding could be difficult to arrange for couples separated by the war. Hastily arranged ceremonies during a leave from the front caused Dorothy Parker to quip, 'It takes two to play a Wedding March – one plays "here comes the bride" the other "there goes the groom".' Certainly weddings were often hurried affairs, yet images of munitions workers wearing their smocks, nurses their veiled uniforms, or of both bride and groom dressed in military uniform, suggest that their officially sanctioned work clothes could seem appropriate and be worn with evident pride.

When there was time to plan, then white or cream wedding dresses were still chosen, though it was not until the Second World War that white weddings were the norm for all classes. The new wartime pared-down silhouette was more economical, using a simple pattern and less fabric, so that dresses could more easily be made at home by a moderately skilled dressmaker. One young working-class British woman working at the Woolwich Arsenal, describes a sister's wedding in 1917 at their London home, with somewhat faint praise:

> She had a white dress and we had dresses with embroidery. Quite a nice little wedding.[12]

Some could afford more elaborately embroidered dresses, heavy with pearl beading and with trains to match. The hair, if not cropped, was still worn up and away from the face, but the veils were lighter, often of tulle or chiffon and sometimes of silver tissue, suggesting something again of the knight's lady. In 1916 and 1917 *Vogue* magazine mentions both shepherdess style gowns and also elaborate medieval dresses with heavy Rapunzel sleeves and jewelled girdle belts worn low on the hip, both showing a desire to escape to an imagined romantic idyll. Fabrics included brocade and panne velvet, as well as more traditional satin. Given the uncertainties of war, it is not surprising that there remained a fashion for the nostalgic, including more corseted dresses, reminding brides of a mother's or grandmother's gown perhaps.

The splendour of regimental dress uniform could be an additional sumptuous element, with its connection to warfare in stark contrast to the waif-like brides. Bridesmaids had until recently tended to be married friends of the bride, but were now more often young, unmarried and dressed similarly to the bride, but with a coloured sash and no veil, often with hair left loose.

For war widows dressing for a second marriage, subdued choices were considered appropriate. Completely white ensembles, even for those who could afford them, might have seemed to ignore a previous marriage. In France in particular, many of the guests, including the bride, might still be in mourning, sometimes for the first husband. Second-time brides were advised to consider dove grey, beige and very pale aqua blue, with only the suggestion of a train, and a modestly truncated veil or small hat instead.

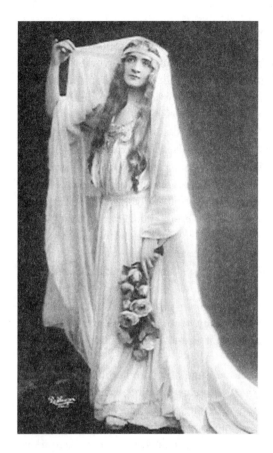

39. Some brides still preferred a romantic idea of dress for their wedding.

Even when marrying for the first time, there was a sense that high-fashion wedding dresses still needed to suggest a certain restraint, given the devastations of the war. The mood was articulated by *Vogue* magazine as 'serious and discreetly gay'. One such bride is described in 'mauve crepe de Chine beaded with crystal and silver, a mauve tulle overdress, and hyacinths in her hair', where hyacinths symbolize constancy and sincerity.[13] In one hastily arranged marriage in 1915 the groom is absent, the French government allowing soldiers to nominate a friend to act for them. The bride is captured on film on the arm of her new husband's proxy, and wearing a plain black suit.[14]

In sum, funerals and mourning clothes are black, but sometimes white; wedding dresses are white, but sometimes black, or at least subdued in colour. Bright, vibrant colour could seem to lack sufficient gravitas for such formal rites of passage.

Identity

Most men killed in action were either buried near to where they fell, or if they died in hospital, in mass military gravesites – Rudyard Kipling's Silent Cities. Due to the nature of the conflict, many bodies were not immediately, if ever, found, and even then it was not always possible to identify individual corpses.

Identity discs proved the best way of keeping track of the vast numbers of fallen soldiers. To wear an ID disc was to recognize their purpose as a means of identification after your death, to be returned to your loved ones as tangible proof, and thus recognizing your own fragile mortality. They had been worn by armies in earlier conflicts, but given the numbers killed in the first months, various attempts were made to improve their design.[15]

Germany was the first country to adopt ID discs, *Erkennungsmarken*, during the Franco-Prussian War of 1870–1, and by September 1915 larger sized oval aluminium discs were issued to allow for more personal information. However, the problem was that when they were removed on death, the body might then be buried in haste, leaving no means of later identification. To solve this problem the information was indented, so that half could be taken and half left with the corpse.

Other belligerents took up either discs that similarly could be broken in two or wore two separate discs. Russia, like Austro-Hungary, provided paper records, which tended to disintegrate after burial. Russian soldiers kept these documents in small wooden phials, but since they were often illiterate, they often discarded them, using their phials for items such as matches instead, so that, all in all, even when properly supplied, they were often unidentifiable after death.

By August 1914 British troops were issued with vulcanized asbestos tags, instead of their initial, more expensive aluminium ones. In British Army parlance, by 1916 'Disc identity, No 2, red' was sent home to relatives to signify an individual's death and another octagonal green disc, 'Disc identity, No 1, green', was intended to remain with the body. Like the problems with paper records and some cheap metal alloys, which tended to corrode, these card ID discs were eventually vulnerable to damp. Moreover, many of the discs were worn on cotton tape or string worn around the neck, which could easily break off in the grave, becoming separated from the body they were intended to identify.

The fear of being anonymous in death drove many soldiers to wear additional tags, made of strong metals, which could be sewn into clothing or worn as bracelets. Yet such sensible purchases must have been sobering and in stark contrast to the fashion accessory they have since become.

Sometimes the only evidence that remained to identify a fallen soldier could be the uniform left behind on the battlefield, seeming to represent the fallen men themselves. Fabric become human form in terrifying metaphor and brute fact:

> Lumps of grey and khaki in every position and still posture, some torn open showing bluish white flesh under broken pink and grey undervests, others bent back and sprawled all ways, gashed, ripped and crumpled.[16]

***

By the end of the war there was an acute awareness of how difficult it would be to identify many of those who had fallen. Survivors had seen for themselves the mangled corpses, the bodies damaged beyond recognition, the vaporizing effects of modern warfare. At home, many families had to be satisfied with the notice that their loved one was missing, presumed dead, and accept that there would be no individual grave to visit.

On Armistice Day 1920 in Paris the remains of a soldier were placed in the *Arc de Triomphe* as *La Tombe du Soldat Inconnu* (the Tomb of the Unknown Soldier). In London a tomb was placed in Westminster Abbey. A newsreel shows the streets full of tens of thousands of silent onlookers as the coffin, draped in a pall and Union flag, processes down Pall Mall, with legions of soldiers, or ex-service people, all in uniform and slow-marching, their heads turned towards the unknown soldier as they pass. In the juddering light of the old cine film, we see that at one point all the men remove their hats as a mark of respect and the sea of heads bow down before this anonymous individual. Across the passage of time there is a palpable sense of their communal grief.

Yet this grieving is not expressed, at least formally, through the clothing of the civilians. When the wreaths are laid, a subtitle describes everyone as wearing black, with the implication that a deliberate choice has been made. And yet, if you compare this extraordinary gathering with that of a joyous occasion at the same period, then there is very much the same balance of predominantly dark clothing, interspersed with lighter coloured coats and jackets. In this context it is not the clothing itself that is meaningful, only the grave manner in which it is worn.

Three years later, Lady Bowes-Lyon married the Duke of York in the Abbey. He wears RAF full dress uniform and she a full length but short-sleeved gown by Madame Handley Seymour, dressmaker to the Queen. It is of the moment, made of ivory chiffon moiré, with horizontal bands of silver lamé, and, significantly perhaps, a train of Flanders lace. Her veil is in a simple Italian medieval style framing her face, and the bodice of her dress is unfitted, held at the hip with a silver girdle, a trail of green tulle and flowers falling to one side and fastened with a jewelled pin – fashionable, sumptuous apparel on a happy occasion. And yet the crowds that gathered to see the couple are mostly darkly dressed, very much as they were at the memorial service in 1920. It was a time of austerity, the memory of the war was still close by, and perhaps darker clothing merited respect, whether in sadness or joy.

Black clothing in itself is beside the point, but rather it is the intention of the wearer through what clothes are available to them that has meaning. Elegant black couture may not necessarily express sincere grief any more than a best coat, which happens to be pale, betokens its absence. However, it is possible, at that royal wedding, to make out details such as bunches of white violets in buttonholes and country bunches adorning hats in the crowd, inexpensive available symbols of romance and hope.

After she was married the then Duchess of York broke with convention by laying her bridal bouquet on the Tomb of the Unknown Soldier, to commemorate her brother Fergus who had died at the Battle of Loos in 1915, in honour of all those other brothers, sons, husbands and fathers who had died throughout the war. This has become the custom ever since, for all royal brides marrying at the abbey. In 2002, Elizabeth II laid her mother's funeral wreath there too.

***

As recently as 2007, a mass gravesite was discovered near Fromelles in France. German troops had dug eight pits during the war for enemy dead, probably after the Battle of Fromelles, or *Fasanenwäldche* (pheasant wood) in 1916.[17] The bodies of Australian and British soldiers were exhumed and eventually reburied by the Commonwealth War Commission. The passage of time had made it impossible to identify many of the bodies. However, both unique artefacts, such as watches and wedding rings found on some of the dead, and DNA samples matched with surviving family members, allowed 75 Diggers of the 5th Australian Division to be indentified, and they were subsequently reinterred in named graves.

9 O BRAVE NEW WORLD

Peace! Thank God for that! It feels very queer too – as if your elastic had snapped.

Edith Appleton, 12 November 1918[1]

Those who survived the war, the wounded, psychologically damaged, or those somehow resilient or lucky enough to find themselves apparently unscathed, and those women for whom the war meant taking their first steps beyond the confines of domestic life, whatever their position and concerns, clothes and all their etceteras still had to be chosen for a life beyond the war. With peace they were thrust back into a work and home life that could seem to disregard the experience they had undergone. It could bring disappointment, particularly for those for whom the war had created a sense of belonging that they had never known before.

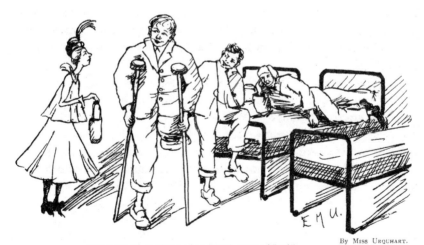

By Miss Urquhart.

"What will you do when you leave hospital, my poor fellow?"
"Oh! I've got a splendid job—in a brewery—making 'ops, and my friend here
he's goin' in for short'and!"

40. A cartoon in *The Fourth*, the magazine of the 4th London Hospital, concerning the rehabilitation of the war-wounded when leaving hospital.

For the victors, peace held hopes of a better future. However catastrophic the war had turned out to be, it had brought people from different classes and nations together. Officers may have taken on the care of their men in the line, but then batmen had reciprocated by taking care of the officers. Women from very different backgrounds had found themselves working alongside each other. For both those who had won and those who had lost, there was a need to adjust to whatever peace might mean. Wearing uniform had helped unite the different organizations of war, and now, in its wake, what effect would a return to civilian clothing bring about?

Under the terms of the Versailles Peace Treaty of June 1919, military uniforms of the defeated armies were destroyed, clothes rent and burnt, and helmets punctured to render them useless. Germany had developed a thorough and efficient demobilization plan to get men quickly out of uniform and back into civilian clothes and employment, but it had been based on an assumption of victory. In the chaos of defeat very little could be done for the returning men. The victorious nations had more reason for optimism, but they too still needed to recover from the expense and trauma of war.

On the Allied side, many kept hold of their uniforms for rough work and possibly for sentiment. It seems likely that some felt reluctant to cast off clothing that they might once have reviled, but had nonetheless been with them throughout the war. A coat, say, that had protected them from the cold, had stood in for bedding, had even taken the place of a stretcher for a wounded comrade.[2]

On demob, soldiers in Britain were sent home in their helmets and uniforms, often in worn and lice-ridden condition, and were then given a choice between a clothing allowance or a plain suit of clothes:

> They gave you a suit, boots ... all the civvy things ... a trilby hat and thoroughly kitted you out. All new clothes. It was a toss up whether you got a good suit or not ... Our greatcoats, we kept.[3]

They were to be given a voucher for £1 to return the greatcoat within 28 days, which could then be cashed at a police station.[4] One British soldier had £1 held back from his war gratuity of £23, payable on return of his coat.[5] In practice, the policy regarding the return of coats and other items was inconsistent and changed as demobilization gathered pace. Another man reported that when he reached Crystal Palace in November 1919, he was surprised not to be allowed to keep his army belt:

> Going through a doorway there was a corporal each side, whipped our tunics open and snatched these belts off.[6]

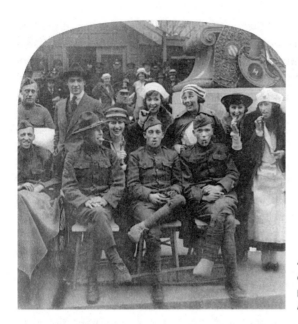

41. A Lollipop Party: wounded doughboys home again, watching a parade with Red Cross nurses, Fifth Avenue, New York, 1919.

The Ordnance Services' Field Service Pocket Book of 1914 laid down that while the majority of a soldier's clothing was deemed 'personal', and therefore his by right, greatcoats and various other items fell into a category that had to be 'returned to store – property of the public'.[7] As the stores became overrun with returns, it was eventually made possible to keep your coat, though since it was public property the £1 charge was made. The Uniform Act of 1894 had forbidden civilians from wearing uniform or parts of uniform, and such prohibitions existed in the majority of participant countries. Apart from the risk of uniforms being misused and variously discredited, wearing uniform in everyday life risked destroying its hard-won mystique.[8]

Women's contribution to the practical business of warfare had, like that of serving men, been symbolized by the wearing of uniform. One question was whether any resulting changes in attitude between the genders could be sustained:

> New forms of patriotism seemed to open the possibility for gender as well as class equality … Yet women in uniform, and especially in khaki, further embodied the fear that the gulf between the sexes … was in danger of eroding, if not disappearing.[9]

Those women who did manage to stay on at their jobs were sometimes reproached for holding on to opportunities that should have been available to the returning men. Cunnington makes the point that, given the fashions of the time, women who did work had to be particularly efficient to justify and maintain their position, but they also had to appear youthful and appealing in their dress. You might say, they were caught in a form of sartorial double bind, for they had to look both sensible and business-like and yet also essentially feminine. Married women were considered by many not to need jobs, because they were classed as dependants of their husbands. A British vicar decries working women as 'showily dressed (fur coats, jewellery), and looking for all the world like flash barmaids'.[10] The reality was that these women had done without the support of men during the long war years, managing their household budgets, feeding and clothing any dependant family, however much they may at times have enjoyed the fripperies available to the independent earner.

It is sometimes said that the war raised women's status, and further, that 'the whole emphasis of a woman's role in society changed'.[11] Yet, in reality, while ideas of female emancipation and greater equality between the sexes had been more fully entertained, very little had changed on the ground in most women's lives. Women who had prayed for the return of their loved ones and had risen to the challenge of war work, were confronted with the reality of what the end of the war meant for their futures. Many lost their better-paid jobs, or found that they no longer had a useful function to fulfil as volunteers, organizing committees, soup kitchens or sewing bees for the troops at home and abroad. Those who had worked in the services, and taken some of the same risks as men, were expected to return to their old domestic roles and poorly paid jobs, or even to a life of leisure without purpose.

There was less need of the lady's maid, when more affluent women had become accustomed to looking after themselves during the war. This meant that together with simpler clothing and less elaborate hairstyles for all, many working-class women who might have considered a domestic post could no longer find a job so easily. There were those who regretted the disruption to the old pre-war social order. The novelist Miss Tennyson Jesse, employed by the British Ministry of Information to report on women workers, was astonished that what she was reluctant to call the 'lower' class, were 'for the most part brought up to think themselves as good as anyone else, and their rights as the chief thing in life'. She reckoned they lacked the 'proper standards of impersonal enthusiasm and imaginative daring which should be the inheritance of us all'.[12]

For men it was no easier, for even when women did make way for them in the workplace, they still had to adjust to being home again. Many had to find

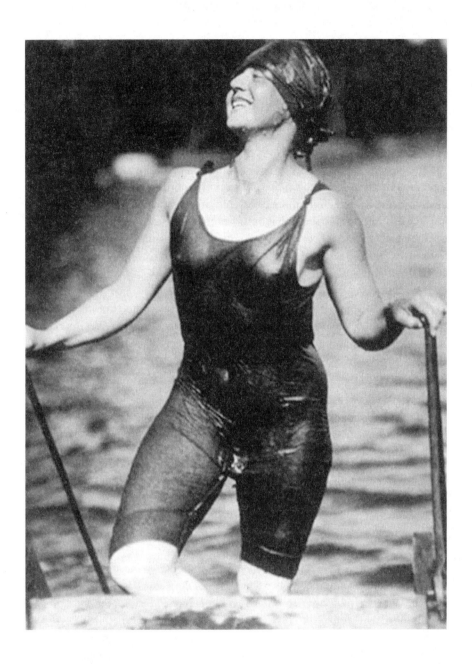

42. A competitive swimmer, 1916, in jersey one-piece suit.

a way of living out their lives with major disabilities. And with peace came anticlimax. The war had been a social as well as a combative experience. The sense of unified purpose was gone, and each individual had to find his or her own way. Men may have longed to be out of uniform, but now their old civilian clothes no longer fitted them as they had imagined they would. They were grown older and leaner perhaps. Often they were very different people now.

The immediate pressures on reunited families could mean that even small freedoms of dress were curtailed, not only by men's expectations of women being appropriately clothed, but because in many cases women no longer had excess income at their disposal. Some regretted the freedom of their wartime uniforms but, conversely, many women seemed happy enough to return to a more cloistered life. However that may be, the idea of women of all classes being independent of male sartorial supervision was no longer an extraordinary idea.

The immediate response to the end of the war was to fall back on pre-war fashions and habits of dress, in a manner of nostalgia for that lost innocence perhaps:

> It almost seemed that Fashion was trying to pick up the thread where it had been interrupted by the war; and many of the day costumes and evening dresses would nearly pass muster for 'pre-war' models of 1913 or '14, with unmistakable hobble effects.[13]

To suggest a clear shift towards more relaxed clothing for women, unhampered by long hair, long skirts, and whalebone and steel corsets, or for men a departure from the gloomy uniformities of post-nineteenth-century dress, is at best a simplification of something that was far more halting in its progress. Anne Hollander resists too lazy a connection being made between the end of hostilities and dress change:

> It is not enough to say that women adopted short skirts after the First World War because they symbolized sexual freedom and permitted easy movement of the legs, since these practical and symbolic effects could have been accomplished in other ways. Some aesthetic reason, some demand internal to the changing look of women and of clothes over quite a long period, required that legs appear just then.[14]

Shorter skirts and more abbreviated underwear for women, and more colourful and less restrictive tailoring for men, were something that evolved gradually, after this initial retreat. What had been lost or at least questioned concerning beliefs, for instance, in a righteous cause, in the power of chivalry, in feminine otherness and the justice of established class systems and expressed in part through dress, was reluctantly faced.

Yet, after a century's hiatus, some men do seem to have become more openly concerned in their own dress, and in its fashionableness. Those who had always been interested, such as the aesthete and the swell, became less marginalized. What film stars and the rich had been wearing during the war became the salient fashion of the times, or at least became a more attainable aspiration. Women's bodies were becoming more exposed to view, and thus their actual rather than imagined forms were laid bare.

More efficient industrial production of fabric and clothing, as a result of the war, meant that lower-income groups could more easily afford mass-produced ready-made clothing. Women who continued to work in secretarial and clerical roles even after marriage, maintained a greater degree of financial independence in regard to dress.[15] What can be said more generally is that the way women dressed underwent a shift to more casual cut and style. This was expressed in detail rather than more obvious change, moving towards the sort of apparently androgynous clothing that is the mark of contemporary fashion, as with such staples as straighter cut masculine-style overcoats and plain shirts.

The aftermath of war could not immediately do away with the consumer frustrations that had been accepted, at least publicly, for patriotic reasons. Advertisements in women's magazines and local newspapers stressed the currency of such expectations, offering 'Peace with Honour' discounts for returning troops, 'Very Special Peace-time Bargains' and reminding all that peace 'only comes ONCE you know, and we want to fittingly celebrate it'. Aware of the lack of resources available, the British drapers Jones and Knight's, for instance, searched for the right approach, promoting 'dainty wearables' but also acknowledging that 'It will no doubt be a Christmas [1918] of really practical gift and giving.'

The expectation that shortages should have been over produced a challenge for the clothing industry. Wartime contracts for uniforms had abruptly come to an end, but then so had the imposed restraints on fashion and shopping:

> Fashion makers, marketers and advertisers were poised to serve the pent-up demand for the new, the modern, and the innovative. Consumerism was about to soar to unprecedented heights in the coming decade.[16]

Women over 30 gained the vote in Britain in 1918, German women in the same year, and in America in 1919, though French women had to wait until 1944. In this respect, the confidence of having the right to vote seems not to have had an appreciable effect on the way women dressed. Despite their political disadvantage, it was Paris and French women who would be at the forefront of changes in dress for women for the next generation. The more adventurous designs coming from Paris failed to find favour in Britain immediately after the war, in that they failed to attract the 'suburban' market, where increasingly the profits were to be made. However, by the end of the decade, hemlines were rising again, and the straight up and down sack dress had become everyday wear for younger women. The conservative tabloid press in Britain could be scathing, referring to the simplified shape as 'designed by a plumber and a cubist meeting in Bedlam'.[17]

Corsets (discussed in Chapter 4) were increasingly set aside, except by older women, with the middle aged increasingly buying the elasticated forms of girdle. The ideal figure for the newly fashionable silhouette was boyish, or *garçonette,* and its simple cut and use of less cloth, benefitted both the home dressmaker and factory production. Stockings were not just black and on occasion white, but came in all colours, more often sugar almond shades, and even as advertised in the *Gazette du Bon Ton* in 1920, in flesh tones, held at the knee with garters. Chest bands or brassieres began to take over from camisoles, in fine cotton and silks. The availability of chemical dyes again, and of artificial fabrics, in particular rayon for both dress fabric and stockings, meant that colourful clothing became more affordable after the dingy colours imposed by the lack of free trade in dyes and fabric during the war.

Fashion would eventually turn towards the appearance of youth, of adolescent slenderness and fitness, leaving middle-aged and older people to their own devices and thus the gulf between young and old deepened. It was the older generation who bore the blame for the war; fashion seemed to be for the young alone. Advertising was beginning to create images of nymph-like creatures to which anyone over 30 would be foolish to aspire. If older women refused to step back, the consequences could be all too cruelly mutton dressed as lamb.

Just as the fashionable woman needed to be boyish, with her breasts battened down if she was unfortunate enough to have them, the fashionable man had to be young and pretty, as if the genders were moving towards each other, towards some androgynous mean. There were attempts to find a unisex form of dress. The Italian futurist Ernesto Michahelles, known as Thayaht, developed a unisex overall *TuTa* in 1919, which he described as 'the most innovative, futuristic garment ever produced in the history of Italian fashion', but apart from a passing fad among the fast set in Florence, it did not catch on.

Some men still young, but who had undergone the carnage of the war, must have found the eager optimism of the 1920s difficult to embrace. After years in uniform, the emphasis on individual expression in clothing might well have seemed alien. Old conformities of dress and manner seemed more fitting, leading many to seem old before their time, wearing again the clothes they remembered their fathers wearing, and refusing to admit a future that seemed to ignore the recent past. Their regimental ties, their wristwatches first worn in the trenches, or the brand of cigarette they had smoked, could be the only apparent evidence that they had been through that war. Moreover those who returned in wheelchairs, burnt or disfigured, in many cases suffering the ongoing effects of shell shock, could not easily adjust to the new, sporty, happy-go-lucky trends, even if they had wanted to.

Older moustachioed men, with bald pates, grey hair and paunches, and who might once have expected their age and status alone to have won them respect, stood no chance of aspiring to the romantic ideal of the age. That said, some older men were beginning to dress with less formality, without risking the sort of negative reaction met by James Keir Hardie when he took up his seat at the House of Commons in the last decade of the nineteenth century, wearing ordinary working men's clothes rather than the customary top hat and tails.

To be on trend, young men wore suits with baggy trousers, with cuffs, and loose, long jackets, often in pale colours that looked best on a muscular but slender frame. Like little boys, they sported Fair Isle sleeveless jumpers over soft-collared button-down shirts, plus fours in snazzy pastel checks ostensibly for the golf course and worn with two-tone shoes with tasselled laces, and figure-hugging jersey suits for sea bathing. They might wear a safari jacket, with long baggy shorts and a cravat at the neck, with long soft leather boots right up to the knee, as if they had just got back from hunting lions in Kenya. Evening wear demanded the casual elegance of single-breasted tuxedos, sometimes in cream for the Riviera look, as the formality of tails was only for older men.

At the beginning of the 1920s, the emphasis was on high-octane hedonism, and now that it was acceptable for women to go about without an escort, parties could be just for young people, brash with cocktails and smoking and high jinks. The trend was for jazz, blues music and dancing the tango, as well as the new, more energetic dances that required both fitness and clothing which could withstand high kicks, like the Black Bottom and later the lindy hop. The charleston dance was first seen in the Ziegfeld Follies musical *Runnin' Wild*, when the athletic style of the African-American dancers was quick to influence the dance halls and nightclubs of the developed world. Flapper shift dresses were short with dropped waist, sometimes just to the knee, with flirty skirts, often fringed, and worn with plain short-sleeved or sleeveless bodices. In the first half of the 1920s they were made in 'droop and drape ... soft fabrics such as lamé, panne velvet and crêpe de Chine, often tied with a deep sash at the hip'.[18] On the head would be worn a broad band with plume attached or jewelled skull cap straight out of the movies, with plain wool felt cloches for daywear, a dab of rouge on each cheek and high pencilled eyebrows like a schoolboy made up as a girl. The new dances incorporated the shimmy move, the shim-me-sha-wabble, where the body is held still while the shoulders undulate.

Hair was at first quite softly bobbed, as with the 'Coconut', or shingled like Clara Bow, but the most severe cut was modelled on the youthful British male style of the Eton crop, very short at the back with a fringe at the front swept back from a side parting. Sometimes short hair was softened by kiss curls in front of the ear, either one on each cheek like the dancer Josephine Baker, or sometimes with a single lock on the forehead – all pasted down with either homemade or commercial gel, or with the aid of dried soup.[19] Victoria Sherrow mentions that these fashionable short haircuts seemed set to destroy the hairnet business, which therefore fought back by pressing for the compulsory use of hairnets in the workplace, whatever the length of hair. However, sales of hairgrips or bobby pins were increased since they were just what was needed to keep a bobbed haircut neatly in place.

Male fashion responded to the flapper with the sheik-look, hoping to smoulder with sex appeal like Rudolph Valentino, with raggedy fur coats, sometimes bell-bottom trousers, wide scarves thrown over the shoulder and hair slicked back with Brilliantine, to become the perfect Latin lover. The origin of this new way of dressing derives from America, so that even in Paris, London and Berlin the atmosphere of illicit excitement that was conjured from Prohibition's speakeasy drinking dens, the wide-boy gangsters in their slick, conspicuously expensive suits and their frivolous-looking girlfriends, seemed to infect nightlife and style more generally.

When the Depression began to take hold at the very end of the 1920s, gangster-style suits had become slimmer in line, and jackets became more fitted. Into the 1930s suits gradually became more wide-shouldered and double-breasted, men seeming to become older with economic adversity. Women's fashion started to evolve towards a more traditional feminine shape, emphasizing the waistline again, and with longer, fuller skirts, and with the breast and cleavage becoming the central focus, supported by more technically sophisticated brassieres. James Laver makes the point that films of the 1920s brought about 'the curious effect of immensely improving women's underwear in real life [with] the abandonment of linen and the substitution of real and artificial silk'.[20]

For those countries that had lost the war, austere economic conditions made interest in clothing and fashion unfeasible, yet its siren call could be a seductive means of escape from the reality of defeat. In Germany, post-war restrictions intensified the atmosphere of decadent refinement in a defeated nation determined to survive. Berlin cabaret vied with the New York speakeasy,[21] American breezy confidence versus sophisticated panache. In German society at large, old school 'class boundaries signified by fashionable attire began to blur' and the idea of the natural nobility of womankind came to the fore, 'based not so much on descent or wealth [but] on individual elegance and distinguished taste'.[22] What was fluid and fanciful in the youthful verve of the flapper in America, solidified into a pre-Second World War female ideal in Germany, athletic, forceful and womanly.

Footage of the time shows the health spas of the late 1920s and '30s and the beginnings of orchestrated mass exercise, where the image is of uniformly fit, well-nourished young men and women, dressed in sensible uniformity. Female hair is neat and there is little evidence of make-up, whereas in the rest of Europe and America an undisguised use of lipstick and mascara was becoming acceptable, certainly in the larger cities. The strong, healthy, no-nonsense image of young German women in these films contains little suggestion of cabaret-style gender play; their figures have full chests, small waists and strapping thighs. Compare this with cabaret's sensual androgynies, of female actors in swaggering male roles, male actors as winsome sirens in bias cut silk velvet and come-hither feathers, and the divergent strands of fashion might be said to betray the mounting tension in society at large. Paul Connerton makes a connection between German mass exercise and the defeat of the war:

> The massed military rallies and gymnastic displays of German fascism were a belated response to the traumatic experience of 1914–18: the legitimating display of fit bodies choreographed in the form of a mass ornament depended for the persuasion of its bodily rhetoric on the never acknowledged but unmistakably present collective memory not only of the many war dead but also, and perhaps even more, of the mutilated bodies of those who had survived the last war but who would no longer be able to form competent elements in a mass ornament shaped out of human bodies.[23]

Coco Chanel was the dominant design influence of the post-war years in Europe and America. The extremes of the frivolous flapper were not for her, preferring to build on her groundbreaking separates, in the context of a new social milieu, of 'smoking cigarettes, drinking cocktails in public [and] driving cars and piloting airplanes'.[24] She had the knack of making the gamin look seem slender and pared down in style, elegant not only for young women but also for the more mature woman. Since it was often older women who had the money for her designs, then this was a significant aspect of her commercial success.

Paul Poiret had been the first to market a perfume under a designer's name (*Rosine* in 1911), but Chanel used simply her name, choosing a clean-cut design of bottle and packaging for her Chanel No 5. It was she who made suntans associated with health and the Riviera lifestyle, rather than the mark of working-class toil,[25] so that women no longer had to be pale to be interesting:

> Sun tans and freckles are affectations which are not only annoying and irritating but which, if not carefully dealt with, may have permanent deleterious effects upon the complexion.[26]

This advice from *The Lady* magazine is not aware that, as with all youth culture, the long-term outcome of sun bathing was hardly the point. The point was to look healthy there and then, and let the future take care of itself.

Chanel's look sported sunglasses, artificial pearls, chic short hair, and svelte, understated cut and dash. The rich of all ages, with the means to afford her, could diet and exercise and not look foolish in her more tailored gear. This was fashion not so much for the young, but one that created an imperative to look youthfully slender, even as the flesh grew older with each passing season. It was not so much youth, but the desire to appear youthful that Chanel helped foster and that has fed the fashion industry ever since.

***

Hasty wartime marriages led to a greater demand for divorce in the 1920s, and therefore more second marriages. Marriage itself was no longer seen as necessarily for life, and this uncertainty provided, from the fashion perspective, a pressure on women to maintain their marriage-ability by maintaining the illusion of lasting youthfulness.

If marriages were breaking up then improved knowledge of and availability of cheaper contraception was called for. From 1920, the development of latex, by the Polish inventor Julius Fromm, meant that condoms were not only thinner and more reliable, but also, because they were more easily mass-produced, more affordable, playing an important role in sexual freedom for both genders.

Anxious for news during the war, people of all classes and across Europe had become accustomed to reading a daily paper, which meant that they had also become more susceptible to advertising. Women's magazines for all income groups had become established, from the cheaper weeklies to aspirational glossy magazines. Now the war was over, companies were unrestrained by national directives towards thrift say, and in America there was commercial radio, further bolstering the desire for new goods.

***

School like military uniform is about control of 'the bodies, minds and even language'.[27] For American, and to some extent British school children when uniform was worn, what came into use after the war was certainly more practical, with simpler cotton dresses and warm wool skirts with button-on straps over the shoulder for girls. Boys wore shorts, and at a later age full-length trousers, though in America young boys tended to wear short trousers buttoned at the knee. Both girls and boys wore knee-length socks, capitalizing on the knitting habit of the war.

These were the children, more comfortably kitted out perhaps, bred on the excitement and drama of the First World War, who would come to fight the next: our parents, grandparents and great-grandparents.

CONCLUSION

This has been a book about appearance. What appearance can reveal about even such a time as the First World War. How what people wore mattered, for the men who fought and those who stayed at home, the women who took up new roles and the children for whom war was all they knew. How clothing and all the minor accessories and trappings associated with dress can be important, and at times have something to say about their broader context.

While women tend to talk about their clothes in letters and diaries, men do so more rarely. Often a soldier in the field will describe his circumstances in detail, his digs, his food, his rifle, and mentions that, for example, his greatcoat is damaged and he is reluctant to wear an alternative because his coat has been with him for two years in the trenches ... and then no more. The resonance of what he means is there, but he does not think it fitting to say more. Clothes have mattered to him, but he does not intend to make a fuss about it.

As I write, there is no one left to talk about their own experience of dress during that First World War. Claude Choules, the last surviving person to see active military service in the war, who also served in the Second World War, died in 2011. At the age of just 14 he became a cadet on the Royal Navy training ship, *Mercury*. The first thing they taught him was 'not ... to handle a sail, wield a cutlass or lay a gun, but ... how to hold a needle and to put his clothes away neatly'.[1] Later he recalls in his memoirs the 'mend and make' sessions on the *Impregnable*, learning how to

> cut a haversack out of coarse duck material and sew it up. Then followed a white flannel shirt and, later, I had to cut out a jumper and a pair of bell-bottomed trousers from six yards of blue serge. We then sewed them up by hand to make a suit of clothes.[2]

Soon he pays someone with a hand-operated sewing machine to make his uniforms, and is promoted to the Captain's galley, where the men are given a new set of clothing every six months, 'so that they always appear very smartly dressed'.

Fast forward to Choules's one hundredth birthday. He is living in Western Australia, and his daughter suggests, since he has enjoyed swimming all his life, that he might like to invest in a new pair of trunks. Habits of thrift learnt during two wars die hard, and he replies:

Oh, I don't know. If I thought I had another 10 years in me it might be worth it.

He lived to the age of 110. He had learnt to understand the importance of dress.

NOTES

Introduction

1 Lyn MacDonald, *1915: The Death of Innocence Interdisciplinary Encounters*. London: Headline, 1993, p. 586.
2 Umberto Eco, cited in John Harvey, *Men in Black*. London: Reaktion Books, 1995, p. 12.
3 Sergeant C. Lippett, 1/8th Battalion, Queen's Royal West Surrey Regiment, 1915, cited in Max Arthur, *Forgotten Voices of the Great War*. London: Ebury Press, 2002.
4 Ibid.
5 Robert Graves, *Goodbye To All That*. London: Penguin, 2011 [1929], p. 77.
6 Ibid., p. 67.
7 'Androgyny is the hallmark of modernity', S. Takeda and K. Spilker, *Fashioning Fashion: European Dress, 1700–1915*. London: Prestel, 2010.
8 Piete Kuhr, Walter Wright, trans. *There We'll Meet Again: A Young German Girl's Diary of the First World War*. London: Walter Wright, 1998 [1982 in German], 4 August 1914.
9 Ibid., 20 July 1915.
10 Corporal G. R. Daniels, 12th Bermondsey Battalion, East Surrey Regiment, cited in MacDonald, *1915: The Death of Innocence*, p. 167.
11 Kuhr, *There We'll Meet Again*, 27 January 1915.
12 Henry Buckle, *A Tommy's Sketchbook: Writings and Drawings from the Trenches*. Stroud: The History Press, 2012, p. 21.
13 Gaston Riou, *The Diary of a French Private: War Imprisonment, 1914–1915*. London: Allen and Unwin, 1916, IWM 14724, POW 1914–15, p. 224.
14 Ernst Jünger, Michael Hofmann trans. *Storm of Steel*. London: Penguin, 2004 [1930 in German], Les Eparges, 1916, p. 26.
15 Gerhard Bauer, personal email, 13 August 2013.
16 *A German Officer's Notebook*, 178th Regiment XII Saxon Corps,1914, IWM 184.
17 Gunnersbury Museum archive, London.
18 Roland Barthes, *The Fashion System*. Berkeley, CA: University of California Press, 1992, p. 11.
19 Pat Barker, *Regeneration*. London: Penguin, 2008 [1991].

Chapter 1: The Prelude

1 Madeline Green, 1884–1947.
2 Juliet Nicolson, *The Perfect Summer: Dancing into Shadow in 1911*. London: John Murray, 2006.

3   *Punch* magazine, 1918.
4   Kate Chopin, *The Awakening and Selected Stories*. Harmondsworth: Penguin, 1984 [1899], p. 58.
5   Lily Bart in Edith Wharton, *The House of Mirth*. Ware: Wordsworth Editions, 2002 [1905], p. 133.
6   Piete Kuhr, *There We'll Meet Again: A Young German Girl's Diary of the First World War*. London: Walter Wright, 1998 [1982 in German], Whit Tuesday, 1918, Schneidemühl, Germany, 80 miles from the Russian front.
7   Gerda Buxbaum, ed., *Icons of Fashion, the 20th Century*. London: Prestel, 2000.
8   Stella Mary Newton, *Health, Art and Reason: Dress Reformers of the 19th Century*. London: John Murray, 1974, p. 155.
9   A. S. Byatt, *The Children's Book*. London: Chatto & Windus, 2009.
10   C. Willett Cunnington, *English Women's Clothing in the Present Century*. London: Faber and Faber, 1952, p. 5.
11   Newton, *Health, Art and Reason*, p. 160.
12   Valerie Steele, *The Corset: A Cultural History*. New Haven, CT: Yale University Press, 2003, p. 64.
13   C. Willett Cunnington, *Why Women Wear Clothes*. London: Faber and Faber, 1941, p. 200.
14   Hew Strachan, *The First World War: A New Illustrated History*. London: Simon and Schuster, 2003, p. 167.
15   Sarah Frantz, *Jane Austen's Heroes and the Great Masculine Renunciation* http://uncfsu.academia.edu/SarahFrantz/Papers/388751, p. 6.
16   W. N. Hodgson, 'England to Her Sons', August 1914.
17   Paul Fussell, *Uniforms: Why We Are What We Wear*. New York: Mariner Books, 2002, p. 6.
18   Gaston Riou, *The Diary of a French Private: War Imprisonment, 1914–1915*. London: Allen and Unwin, 1916, IWM 14724, pp. 35–6.
19   The invention of the trouser press in 1890s made this easier to achieve for those without a manservant.
20   Edward VII adopted the hat after a visit to Bad Homburg in Germany, which influenced many to follow his lead.
21   Cunnington, *English Women's Clothing*, p. 140.
22   Jane Robinson, *Bluestockings: The Remarkable Story of the First Women to Fight for an Education*. London: Profile, 2009, p. 134.
23   Stefan Zweig, *The World of Yesterday*. London: Pushkin Press, 2011 [1943], part IX, The First Hours of the War of 1914.
24   Kuhr, *There We'll Meet Again*, 2 August 1914.
25   James Laver, in *A Concise History of Costume*. London: Thames and Hudson, 1969, p. 229, suggests that 'the war, in fact, as all wars do, had a deadening effect on fashion, and there is little to record until the conflict is over'.
26   Nosheen Khan, *Women's Poetry of the First World War*. Lexington, KY: University of Kentucky, 1988, p. 11.

Chapter 2: Uniform, Chivalry and Doing One's Bit

1   Malcolm Brown, *The Imperial War Museum Book of The First World War*. London: Guild Publishing, 1991 p. 40.
2   Clifton J. and Charles Cameron Cate, *Notes: A Soldier's Memoir of World War One*. Victoria, BC: Trafford, 2005. pp. 100–1.

3   Paul Fussell, *Uniforms: Why We Are What We Wear.* New York: Mariner Books, 2002, p. 34.

4   John Harvey, *Men in Black.* London: Reaktion Books, 1995, p. 19.

5   Ibid., p. 14.

6   Smokeless powder was first used in the 1880s – making it far easier to hit one's target.

7   http://www.1914-1918.be/insolite_dernier.

8   Toni Pfanner, 'Military Uniforms and the Law of War', *IRRC,* March 2004, vol. 86, no. 853, p. 98.

9   Ibid., p. 223.

10 A high-necked, long-sleeved partial blouse, that ends just below the bust, held in place by tapes, and particularly useful before the advent of effective deodorants.

11 The raven was thought to be unusually intelligent and crafty.

12 Karen Hagemann and Stefanie Schüler-Springorum, eds, *Home Front: The Military, War and Gender in Twentieth Century Germany.* Oxford: Berg, 2002, p. 47.

13 Gerhard Bauer, personal email, 13 August 2013.

14 The spelling of 'Welch' was widely used but unofficial until 1920.

15 Robert Graves, *Goodbye To All That.* London: Penguin, 2011 [1929], p. 86.

16 John Mollo, *Military Fashion: A Comparative History of the Uniforms of the Great Armies of the Seventeenth Century to the First World War.* London: Barrie and Jenkins, 1972, p. 227.

17 Lyn Allyn and Clarence A. Bush, *Love from Chezeaux: WWI Memoirs of Clarence Bush.* Bloomington, IN: Author House, 2006, p. 49.

18 Hew Strachan, *The First World War: A New Illustrated History.* London: Simon and Schuster, 2003, p. 162.

19 Mannie Gentile's combathelmets.blogspot.com, Museum of America, 2009.

20 Gerhard Bauer, personal email, 13 August 2013.

21 Kaiser Wilhelm wore one such when visiting Istanbul in 1917. Cited in http://landships.info.

22 Sabina Brändli in *Von schneidigen Offizieren,* cited in Hagemann and Schüler-Springorum, eds, *Home Front,* p. 199.

23 F. G. H. Garrett of 3rd Light Horse Infantry AIF, diary entry dated 1 June 1915. www.grantsmilitaria.com.

24 Niall Ferguson, *The Pity of War.* London: Allen Lane, 1998, p. 350.

25 Oswald Croft, British NCO with 5th Battalion Seaforth Highlanders, La Chapelle, 1914, IWM 4440.

26 Harold Joseph Hayward, 12th Battalion Gloucestershire Regiment, 1914–16, officer 15th Battalion Welsh Regiment on WF 1918, IWM 9422.

27 Pfanner, 'Military Uniforms', p. 105.

28 Peter Englund, ed., *The Beauty and the Sorrow: An Intimate History of the First World War.* London: Profile, 2011, p. 175.

29 Janet Flanner, *Paris was Yesterday 1925–39.* New York: Penguin, 1979, p. 126.

30 Pat Shipman, *Femme Fatale: Love, Lies and the Unknown Life of Mata Hari.* New York: HarperCollins, 2007, p. 450.

31 Private Papers of Sister Cecile, 1914–18, IWM 6807.

32 Carl Zuckmayer, *Der Hauptmann von Köpenick,* 1931.

33 Vera Brittain, *Testament of Youth.* London: Virago, 1988 [1933], p. 114.

34 Fussell, *Uniforms,* p. 24.

35 Henry Williamson, *The Patriot's Progress.* Stroud: Sutton, 2004 [1930], p. 19.

36 Philipp Witkop, *German Students' War Letters.* Philadelphia, PA: Pine Street Books, 2013, p. 344.

37 Walter Ambroselli, ibid., 19 January 1915, p. 187.

38   Harold Joseph Hayward, 12th Battalion Gloucestershire Regiment, WF 1914–16, officer 15th Battalion Welch Regiment, WF 1918, IWM 9422.

39   Evangeline Booth and Grace Livingston Hill, *The War Romance of the Salvation Army*. London: J. B. Lippincott, 1919, p. 48.

40   J. W. Palmer, Royal Field Artillery, in Max Arthur, *Forgotten Voices of the Great War*. London: Ebury Press, 2002, p. 31.

41   Sergeant F. G. Udall, Royal Fusiliers, ibid., p. 249.

42   Graves, *Goodbye To All That*, p. 109.

43   Ferguson, *The Pity of War*, p. 350.

44   Wilhelm His, *A German Doctor at the Front*. Washington DC: The National Service Publishing Company, 1933, p. 14.

45   'For the Well Dressed Man', *Vanity Fair*, October 1918.

46   *Harper's Bazar*, 1918, http://www.oldmagazinearticles.com/ww1_women_uniforms.

47   Billy Prior, in Pat Barker, *Regeneration*. London: Penguin, 2008 [1991], p. 66.

48   Sandy Arbuthnot, in John Buchan, *Greenmantle*. Oxford: World Classics, 1993 [1916], p. 8.

49   Williamson, *Patriot's Progress*, p. 11.

50   Charles Peck, *Allen Peck's WWI Letters Home, 1917–1919: US Army Pilot Assigned to France*. New York, NY: iUniverse, 2005, 1 September 1918.

51   Harold Joseph Hayward 1914, IWM 9422.

52   Lyn MacDonald, *1915: The Death of Innocence*. London: Headline, 1993, p. 153.

53   G. R. Daniels, ibid., 12th Bermondsey Battalion, East Surrey Regiment.

54   Henry Buckle, *A Tommy's Sketchbook: Writings and Drawings from the Trenches*. The History Press, 2012, 1914, p. 25.

55   Graves, *Goodbye To All That*, La Bourse, 22 May 1915, p. 110.

56   W. Worrell, Rifleman, summer 1917, cited in Lyn MacDonald, *They Called it Passchendaele: The Story of the Third Battle of Ypres and of the Men who Fought in it*. London: Penguin, 1993 [1978], p. 80.

57   Piete Kuhr, *There We'll Meet Again: A Young German Girl's Diary of the First World War*. London: Walter Wright, 1998 [1982 in German] 30 August 1918.

58   Ibid., 8 November 1918. Piete Kuhr did become a dancer and performed this dance in 1933 in Berlin.

59   Gaston Riou, *The Diary of a French Private: War Imprisonment, 1914–1915*. London: Allen and Unwin, 1916, IWM 14724, Bavarian fortress, 1914–15, pp. 107–8.

60   Group Captain Frederick Winterbottom, 29th Squadron Royal Flying Corps, POW 1917–18, IWM 7462, reel 2.

61   Ibid., p. 282–3.

62   Strachan, *The First World War*, p. 165.

63   Staff Sergeant James Kain, Army Ordnance Corps, cited in Lyn MacDonald, *Somme*. London: Penguin, 1983, p. 201.

64   Erich Maria Remarque, *All Quiet on the Western Front*. London: Vintage, 1996 [1929], p. 16.

65   Ibid., p. 31.

66   His, *A German Doctor at the Front*, p. 106.

67   William Thomas Cowley, NCO with 11th Coy Army Service Corps, Chocolate Hill, 1915, IWM 8866.

68   Mary Ludlum's diary, cited in Lyn MacDonald, *The Roses of No Man's Land*. Harmondsworth: Penguin, 1993 [1980], p. 34.

69   Lorna Neill, cited in Susan R. Grayzel, *Women's Identities at War: Gender, Motherhood and Politics in Britain and France during the First World War*. Chapel Hill, NC: University of North Carolina Press, 1999, p. 205.

70   Ibid., p. 272.

71   Glenn E. Hyatt, *Fredericksburg Area Military History and Collectors' Association*, http://members.tripod.com/-Fbg_mem_museum/unitalk/unipart1.htm.
72   Peck, *Allen Peck's WWI Letters Home*, 6 July 1917.
73   *The Great War*, BBC television documentary, 1964.
74   The Flieger Abteilung Bavarian Flying Unit, 1917.
75   Mollo, *Military Fashion*, p. 207.
76   Remarque, *All Quiet on the Western Front*, p. 40.
77   Claire M. Tylee, *The Great War and Women's Consciousness*. Iowa City: University of Iowa Press, 1990, p. 197.
78   Robert Service, 'Over the Parapet', 1916.
79   Rose Macaulay, 'Many Sisters to Many Brothers', in Helen Zenna Smith, ed., *Not So Quiet: Stepdaughters of War*. New York: The Feminist Press CUNY, 1978 [1930], p. 252.
80   Fussell, *Uniforms*, p. 202, also here referring to academic uniform.
81   Norman Stone, *World War One: A Short History*. New York: Basic Books, 2009, p. 5.
82   Witkop, *German Students' War Letters*, p. 344.
83   Siegfried Sassoon, 'Glory of Women', 1918.
84   Peck, *Allen Peck's WWI Letters Home*, 22 November 1917.
85   Walter Dean Myers and Bill Miles, *The Harlem Hellfighters*. London: HarperCollins, 2006, p. 61.
86   Ibid., p. 147.
87   Margaret Jean Hay, 'Changes in Clothing and Struggles over Identity in Colonial Western Africa', in Jean Allman, ed., *Fashioning Africa: Power and the Politics of Dress*. Bloomington, IN: Indiana University Press, 2004, p. 68.
88   Private Shuttleworth, BASC, 1915, cited in Arthur, *Forgotten Voices*.
89   Valerie Cumming, *Understanding Fashion History*. London: Batsford, 2011, p. 103.

Chapter 3: Men in Civvies; Women in Uniform

1   Michel Corday, in Peter Englund, ed., *The Beauty and the Sorrow: An Intimate History of the First World War*. London: Profile, 2011, p. 282.
2   Kendra van Cleave, 'Fashion', in James Ciment and Thadeus Russell, *The Home Front Encyclopedia: United States, Britain and Canada in World War I and II*. Santa Barbara: ABC-CLIO, 2006, pp. 312–3.
3   Will Ellsworth-Jones, *We Will Not Fight: The Untold Story of World War One's Conscientious Objectors*. London: Aurum Press, 2008.
4   Mrs Barstow was the writer Baroness Orczy, author of that archetypal man of modest courage, the Scarlet Pimpernel, who fought his war not in uniform at all, but in the gorgeous guise of a fop.
5   Robin MacDonald, 'White Feather Feminism: The recalcitrant progeny of radical suffragist and conservative pro-war Britain', Fort Myers, FL: Florida Gulf Coast University, 1998 http://itech.fgcu.edu/&/issue1/feather.htm.
6   Private Harold Carter, 1915, in Max Arthur, *Forgotten Voices of the Great War*. London: Ebury Press, 2002.
7   Jane Cox, IWM 705.
8   Helen Hamilton in Nosheen Khan, *Women's Poetry of the First World War*. Lexington, KY: University of Kentucky, 1988, p. 80.
9   Roland Barthes, *The Fashion System*. Berkeley, CA: University of California Press, 1992, p. 11.
10 Sarah Macnaughton, 20 September 1914, in Englund, ed., *The Beauty and the Sorrow*, p. 25.

11   Claudia Brush Kidwell, 'Gender Symbols or Fashion Details', in Claudia Brush Kidwell and Valerie Steele, eds., *Men and Women*, cited in John Harvey, *Men in Black*. London: Reaktion Books, 1995, p. 16.

12   Gregory Anderson, ed., *White Blouse Revolution: Female Office Workers since 1870*. Manchester: Manchester University Press, 1988, p. 43.

13   Lyn MacDonald, *1915: The Death of Innocence*. London: Headline, 1993, pp. 231–2.

14   Piete Kuhr, *There We'll Meet Again: A Young German Girl's Diary of the First World War*. London: Walter Wright, 1998 [1982 in German], 17 March 1918.

15   Gaston Riou, *The Diary of a French Private: War Imprisonment, 1914–1915*. London: Allen and Unwin, 1916, IWM 14724, *Pantalons rouges*, or the red-trousered ones, was a nickname used for French soldiers even after the changeover to khaki, p. 90.

16   Cheryl Buckley, 'De-Humanized Females and Amazonians: British wartime fashion and its representation in *Home Chat*, 1914–1918', in *Gender and History*. Oxford: Blackwell, November 2002, vol. 14, no. 3, p. 516.

17   Ibid., p. 525, extract from *Home Chat*, 10 October 1914.

18   Amy Elizabeth May, IWM 684.

19   Florence Cordell, Museum of Transport Archive.

20   IWM EPH 5093.

21   Fashion article after the battle of the Marne 1914, cited in C. Willett Cunnington, *English Women's Clothing in the Present Century*. London: Faber and Faber, 1952, p. 121.

22   Angela Olivia Limerick, VAD St Mary's Hospital Paddington, London, IWM 377.

23   Ibid.

24   Working-class women had always had to contribute their labour to survive. In Britain, for example, domestic service held its ground, numbers dropping from 1,658,000 at the beginning of the war to a still sizeable 1,258,000 in 1918. Statistics in Arthur Marwick, *The Deluge: British Society and the First World War*. London: Macmillan, 2006 [1965].

25   Bianca Schönberger, 'Motherly Heroines and Adventurous Girls' in Karen Hagemann and Stefanie Schüler-Springorum, eds, *Home Front: The Military, War and Gender in Twentieth Century Germany*. Oxford: Berg, 2002, p. 87.

26   Cited in Lyn MacDonald, *The Roses of No Man's Land*. Harmondsworth: Penguin, 1993 [1980], p. 73.

27   Lindy Woodhead, *War Paint: Elizabeth Arden and Helena Rubenstein, their Lives, their Times, their Rivalry*. London: Virago, 2003, p. 107.

28   'The BF' in Helen Zenna Smith, ed., *Not So Quiet: Stepdaughters of War*. New York: The Feminist Press CUNY, 1978 [1930].

29   Ibid., p. 25.

30   Anne Powell, *Women in the War Zone: Hospital Service in the First World War*. Stroud: The History Press, 2001, Military Hospital, Warsaw 1914.

31   H. de Watteville, 'The Royal Army Clothing Department', in *RUSI Journal*, 1932, vol. 77, issue 507.

32   The disabling hobble skirt did remain an evening wear fashion.

33   Hagemann and Schüler-Springorum, eds, *Home Front*, p. 94.

34   Alice Salomon in *Charakter*, cited ibid., p. 99.

35   Valerie Cumming, in *Understanding Fashion History* (London: Batsford, 2011), discusses how smocks had been adopted a generation before by the Aesthetic Movement as 'symbols of simplicity and honest labour' (p. 105) and it is likely that some of this association remained.

36   Moira Donald and Linda Hurcombe, eds, *Representations of Gender from Prehistory to the Present*. London: Macmillan, 2000, p. 200.

37   Angela Woollacott, 'Dressed to Kill', in ibid., p. 202.

NOTES

38 *Daily Express*, 27 November 1916, cited in Joyce Marlow, ed., *The Virago Book of Women and the Great War*. London: Virago, 2005 [1998], p. 173.
39 Ian Beckett, *Home Front, 1914–1918: How Britain Survived the Great War*. The National Archives, 2006, p. 88.
40 Caroline Playne, 1931, cited in Buckley, 'De-Humanized Females', p. 522.
41 Amy Elizabeth May, IWM 684.
42 Marlow, ed., *Women and the Great War*, p. 85.
43 Georgetown Filling Factory, Glasgow, cited in Donald and Hurcombe, *Representations of Gender*, p. 23.
44 Ibid., Elizabeth Gore, Woolwich Arsenal, p. 165.
45 Cited in Angela Woollacott, *On Her Their Lives Depend: Munitions Workers in the Great War*. Berkeley, CA: University of California Press, 1994, p. 22.
46 Madeline Ida Bedford, 'Munition Wages', in Catherine Reilly, ed., *Scars Upon My Heart: Women's Poetry and Verse of the First World War*. London: Virago, 1981, p. 7.
47 Joyce Eileen Eames, IWM 11719, 13 years old in 1918.
48 'Munitions Work' by Naomi Loughnan, in Marlow, ed., *Women and the Great War*, pp. 166–7.
49 Buckley, 'De-Humanized Females', p. 525.
50 Ibid., p. 518.
51 C. Willett Cunnington, *Why Women Wear Clothes*. London: Faber and Faber, 1941, p. 193.
52 Elizabeth Ewing, *Women in Uniform through the Centuries*. London: Batsford, 1975, p. 90.
53 *Observer* Women's Page, 13 December 1914.
54 Annie Sarah Edwards, IWM 740.
55 Ibid.
56 Ibid.
57 Marwick, *The Deluge*, 30 August 1916.
58 Sinéad McCoole, *No Ordinary Women: Irish Female Activists in the Revolutionary Years, 1900–1923*. Dublin: The O'Brien Press, 2003, p. 31.
59 Anne Haverty, in Marlow, ed., *Women and the Great War*, p. 225.
60 Gunnersbury Museum record of uniform of H. O. C. Smith, who joined the WLA in 1918.
61 Beckett, *Home Front, 1914–1918*.
62 Rose Dorrie, British Library 29322.
63 Lilian Wyles 1919, cited in Ewing, *Women in Uniform*, p. 100.
64 *Daily Mail*, 30 March 1915.
65 *The Globe*, 21 July 1916.
66 Susan R. Grayzel, *Women's Identities at War: Gender, Motherhood and Politics in Britain and France during the First World War*. Chapel Hill, NC: University of North Carolina Press, 1999, p. 20, B. Hopkins, 'WVR Midland: Uniform, its meaning and how it should be worn', 1915.
67 Paul Fussell, *Uniforms: Why We Are What We Wear*. New York: Mariner Books, 2002, p. 156.
68 Irene Schuessler Poplin, 'Nursing uniforms: Romantic idea, functional allure or instrument of social change?', in *Nursing History Review 2*, 1994, p. 155.
69 Oberin Anna von Zimmermann, cited in Hagemann and Schüler-Springorum, eds, *Home Front*, p. 89.
70 Miss Ethel Jones was a nursing sister in the APMMC, serving in Birmingham's Southern General Hospital. She was issued with the sum of £2 every six months for uniform, but if anyone left the Corps within three months of a payment being issued, then they were required to repay £1. NationalArchives.gov.uk/womeninuniform/almeric_paget.profile.
71 Lorna Neill's journal, February 1916, *Cantine Anglaise*, in MacDonald, *The Roses of No Man's Land*, p. 100.

72   Princess Marie de Croy, cited in Ewing, *Women in Uniform*, p. 88.

73   Terri Arthur, *Fatal Decision: Edith Cavell, World War One Nurse*. Milpitas: Beagle Books, 2011, p. 299.

74   Mabel Bone, cited in Lyn MacDonald, *The Roses of No Man's Land*, p. 110.

75   Coningsby Dawson, *The Glory of the Trenches*, https://archive.org/stream/gloryoftrenches00daws

76   Cited in Grayzel, *Women's Identities at War*, p. 193.

77   Powell, *Women in the War Zone*, p. 70.

78   Yvonne McEwen, *It's a Long Way to Tipperary*, p. 75.

79   Kit Dodsworth, cited in MacDonald, *The Roses of No Man's Land*, p. 78.

80   Grayzel, *Women's Identities at War*, p. 283.

81   MacDonald, *The Roses of No Man's Land*, p. 81.

82   Cited in Anne Powell, *Women Doctors and Nurses on the Western and Eastern Fronts During the First World War*, http://www.millicentsutherlandambulance.com

83   Cited in Powell, *Women in the War Zone*, p. 108.

84   Florence Farnborough, Moscow, 12 February 1915, in Englund, ed., *The Beauty and the Sorrow*, p. 84.

85   Vera to Edward Brittain, Imtarfa Hospital, Malta, 10 October 1916, in Alan Bishop and Mark Bostridge, eds, *Letters from a Lost Generation: First World War Letters of Vera Brittain and Four Friends*. London: Abacus, 1998.

86   Vera Brittain, *Testament of Youth*. London: Virago, 1988 [1933], p. 328.

87   Evangeline Booth and Grace Livingston Hill, *The War Romance of the Salvation Army*. London: J. P. Lippincott, 1919, p. 157.

88   Ibid., p. 16.

89   Bernard Finn and Barton C. Hacker, *Materializing the Military*. Washington DC: The Smithsonian Institution, 2005, p. 71.

90   Alison Lurie, *The Language of Clothes*. London: Bloomsbury, 1992 [1981], p. 219: 'It is a universal rule that when clothes are uncomfortable, high-status clothes will be more uncomfortable'.

91   Kate Adie, *Corsets to Camouflage: Women and War*. London: Hodder and Stoughton, 2003, p. 38.

92   Richard Holmes, *Tommy: The British Soldier on the Western Front 1914–1918*. London: Harper Perrennial, 2004, p. 255.

93   Ibid.

94   *Home this Afternoon*, British Library ILP0168195, BBC 30911.

95   'So boldly did I fight me boys although I'm but a wench/ and in buttoning up me trousers so often have I smiled/ to think I lay with a thousand men and a maiden all the while', Steeleye Span, 'Female Drummer', *Individually and Collectively*, 1972.

96   *Morskaia*, the Russian for 'naval', adopted as a *nom de guerre*.

97   Louise Miller, *A Fine Brother: The Life of Captain Flora Sandes*. London: Alma Books, 2012, p. 273.

Chapter 4: The Fabric and Furbelows

1   A. J. Mills, F. Godfrey and B. Scott, 'Take Me Back To Dear Old Blighty', British wartime song, 1916.

2   Ella Potato whose 'chief worry in life is the fear of losing her hairpins', Helen Zenna Smith, ed., *Not So Quiet: Stepdaughters of War*. New York: The Feminist Press CUNY, 1978 [1930], p. 28.

3   Erich Maria Remarque, *All Quiet on the Western Front*. London: Vintage, 1996, p. 7.

4   Archie Surfleet, 13th East Yorkshire Regiment, http://www.sparticus.schoolnet.co.uk/ FWWlatrines.htm, ibid.

5   Guy Chapman, *Vain Glory*, cited ibid.

6   Ruth Cowen, ed., *War Diaries, A Nurse at the Front: The First World War Diaries of Sister Edith Appleton*. London: IWM and Simon and Schuster, 2012, p. 34.

7   Evangeline Booth and Grace Livingston Hill, *The War Romance of the Salvation Army*. London: J. B. Lippincott, 1919 p. 203.

8   C. Willett Cunnington, *Why Women Wear Clothes*. London: Faber and Faber, 1941, p. 251.

9   Crosbie Garstin, 'Chemin des Dames', written during the action of the Battle of Chemin des Dames, 1917.

10   Cowen, ed., *The First World War Diaries of Sister Edith Appleton*, p. 56.

11   Frances Osborne, *The Bolter: Idina Sackville – The Woman who Scandalised 1920s Society and Became White Mischief's Infamous Seductress*. London: Virago, 2008, p. 64.

12   Sebastian Faulks, *Birdsong*, cited in John Mullan, *Guardian*, 22 June 2012.

13   Philip Ollerenshaw, 'Textile business in Europe during the First World War 1914–1918', Business History, January 1999, vol. 41, issue 1, p. 8.

14   Ibid., p. 5.

15   Lawrence James, *Warrior Race: A History of the British at War*. London: Abacus, 2001, p. 516.

16   Jessie Arrowsmith, textile worker in Batley and Leeds, IWM 723.

17   Harry Bashford, NCO with Bedfordshire and Hertfordshire Regiment, Western Front 1916–18, IWM 9987.

18   Lyn MacDonald, *1915: The Death of Innocence*. London: Headline, 1993, p. 153.

19   Diana Epstein, *The Button Book*. London: Running Press, 1996, p. 87.

20   Mark Benedict, *On the Home Front*, www.reenactor.net.

21   Grace Lovat Fraser, *Textiles by Britain*. London: Allen and Unwin, 1948, p. 96.

22   *The Reading Eagle*, 16 September 1917.

23   Piete Kuhr, *There We'll Meet Again: A Young German Girl's Diary of the First World War*. London: Walter Wright, 1998 [1982 in German], 28 January 1915.

24   Sister Cecile, IWM 97/27.

25   Harry Carlton and Joe Tunbridge, 1915.

26   *Navy and Army Illustrated*, 2 September 1899, cited in John Mollo, *Military Fashion*. London: Barrie and Jenkins, 1972, p. 228.

27   C. Willett Cunnington, *English Women's Clothing in the Present Century*. London: Faber and Faber, 1952, p. 31.

28   Mollo, *Military Fashion*, p. 211.

29   Ibid., p. 218.

30   Kenneth Page, 40 Brigade, Royal Field Artillery, cited in Lyn MacDonald, *Somme*. London: Penguin, 1983, 25 June 1916, p. 52.

31   George Pocock, 9th Battalion Welch Regiment, IWM 9761.

32   Remarque, *All Quiet on the Western Front*, p. 7.

33   Charles Peck, *Allen Peck's WWI Letters Home, 1917–1919: US Army WWI Pilot Assigned to France*. New York, NY: iUniverse, 2005, 21 November 1917.

34   William Bernard Whitmore, 14th Service Battalion, Royal Warwickshire Regiment, 3 September 1915. www.firstworldwar.com/diaries/whitmore.

35   George Pocock, IWM 9761, village near Loos, see note 31 above.

36   Rafael de Nogales, July 1916, in Peter Englund, ed., *The Beauty and the Sorrow: An Intimate History of the First World War*. London: Profile, 2011, p. 278.

37   Albert 'Smiler' Marshall, 1st Battalion Essex Yeomanry, in Max Arthur, *Last Post*. London. Weidenfeld & Nicolson, 2005, p. 46.

38 Frederick Charles Higgins, NCO 4th Battalion Royal Fusiliers, Western Front 1915–17, IWM 9884.
39 Cynthia Crossen, 'Women, smoking, share checkered history', *The Wall Street Journal*, in *Chicago Tribune*, 12 March 2008.
40 *The Washington Post*, 1914, ibid.
41 Lindy Woodhead, *War Paint: Elizabeth Arden and Helena Rubenstein, their Lives, their Times, their Rivalry*. London: Virago, 2003, p. 107.
42 Cited in Susan R. Grayzel, *Women's Identities at War: Gender, Motherhood and Politics in Britain and France during the First World War*. Chapel Hill, NC: University of North Carolina Press, 1999, p. 43.
43 Rafael de Nogales, 13 February 1916, in Englund, ed., *The Beauty and the Sorrow*, p. 222.
44 Ralph Bell, cited in Tim Cook, 'Rum in the Trenches', *Legion Magazine*, 1 September 2002, http://legionmagazine.com/en/2002/09/rum-in-the-trenches.
45 Ernest Spillett, 46th Battalion, letter home, 1917, cited ibid.
46 Steve Humphries and Richard van Emden, *All Quiet on the Home Front: An Oral History of Life in Britain during the First World War*. London: Headline, 2004, p. 236.
47 Stephen McGreal, *The War on Hospital Ships, 1914–1918*. Barnsley: Pen and Sword Maritime, 2008, p. 116.
48 A claim made by Charles Nessler who invented the permanent wave and might be said to have had an interest in women maintaining a certain length of hair.
49 Olive King, Salonica, 20 July 1916, in Englund, ed., *The Beauty and the Sorrow*, p. 279.
50 Aileen Ribiero, *Dress and Morality*. London: Batsford, 1986, p. 154.
51 Caroline Cox, *Good Hair Days: A History of British Hairdressing*. London: Quartet, 1999, p. 38.
52 Maria Botchkareva, cited in Christine Hatt, *The First World War, 1914–18*. London: Evans Brothers, 2000, p. 30.
53 Victoria Sherrow, *Encyclopedia of Hair: A Cultural History*. Westport CT: Greenwood Press, 2006, p. 66.
54 Kuhr, *There We'll Meet Again*, 17 August 1914.
55 Cunnington, *English Women's Clothing*, p. 133.
56 Anne Powell, *Women Doctors and Nurses on the Western and Eastern Fronts during the First World War*. http://www.millicentsutherlandambulance.com.
57 28 March 1918, cited in Arthur Marwick, *The Deluge: British Society and the First World War*. London: Macmillan, 2006 [1965], p. 229.
58 Lyn Woodhead, *War Paint*, p. 106.
59 MacDonald, *Somme*. London: Penguin, 1983, p. 80.
60 Denyse Beaulieu, *The Perfume Lover: A Personal History of Scent*. London: HarperCollins 2012, p. 73.
61 Alexander Stewart, *The Experiences of a Very Unimportant Officer*. London: Hodder, 2009, 2 June 1916, p. 56.
62 Norman Stone, *World War One: A Short History*. New York: Basic Books, 2009, p. 111.
63 Ibid., p. 42.
64 Cowen, ed., *The First World War Diaries of Sister Edith Appleton*, pp. 221 and 185.
65 Smith, ed., *Not So Quiet*, p. 20.
66 Harold Bashford, British NCO, Bedfordshire and Hertfordshire Regiment, Western Front 1916–18, IWM 9987.
67 Henry Buckle, *A Tommy's Sketchbook: Writings and Drawings from the Trenches*. Stroud: The History Press, 2012, p. 25.
68 Lieutenant Edwin Evan Jones, signaller with Royal Garrison Artillery, private papers of Edwin Jones, IWM documents 15429, 21 January and 14 June 1916.
69 Henry Williamson, *The Patriot's Progress*. Stroud: Sutton, 2004 [1930], p. 79.

NOTES

70   Cited in Arthur Marwick, *The Great War – and Modern Memory*. Oxford University Press, 1975, p. 300.
71   Albert Hurst, 17th Battalion, Manchester Regiment, October 1915, Suzanne, IWM 11582.
72   Gaston Riou, *The Diary of a French Private: War Imprisonment, 1914–1915*. London: Allen and Unwin, 1916, IWM 14724, 20 May 1915, p. 280.
73   Ibid., 21 October 1914, p. 151.
74   Otto Braun, *The Diary of Otto Braun: With Selections of his Letters and Poems*. London: Heinemann, 1924, 9 June 1915.
75   Frederick Charles Goodman, 2/1st London Field Ambulance, Royal Army Medical Corps, Western Front 1916–18, IWM 9398.
76   Thomas McIndoe, 12th Battalion Middlesex Regiment, Western Front 1914–15, IWM 568.
77   Frederick Charles Goodman, IWM 9398.
78   Christine Hope, 'Caucasian Female Body Hair and American Culture', in *Journal of American Culture*, 2004, vol. 5, issue 1.
79   J. A. Sommerville, Australian Imperial Force war diaries, 16 June 1918.
80   Kate Adie, *Corsets to Camouflage: Women and War*. London: Hodder and Stoughton, 2003, p. 68.
81   Private Allen, Yorkshire ATS, collection of the Women's Royal Army Corps Museum, now transferred to the National Army Museum.
82   Stephanie Pedersen, *Bra: A Thousand Years of Style, Support and Seduction*. Newton Abbot: David and Charles, 2004.
83   Valerie Steele, *The Corset: A Cultural History*. New Haven, CT: Yale University Press, 2003, p. 151.
84   J. Sanders Department Store, *Ealing and Hanwell Post*, 7 and 14 March 1914.
85   Edmund Blunden, *Undertones of War*. London: Penguin, 2000, p. 127.
86   They were, however, issued to the British Land Army in WWII.
87   *Mémorial de Verdun*, French museum dedicated to the First World War.
88   Marcel Proust, *Remembrance of Things Past: vol III: Time Regained*. London: Chatto & Windus, p. 744, cited in Elizabeth Wilson, *Adorned in Dreams: Fashion and Modernity*. London: Virago, 1985, p. 188.
89   Genesis 31:49.
90   Denise van Patten, www.collectdolls.about.com.
91   Lyn MacDonald, *1915: The Death of Innocence*, p. 4.
92   Kuhr, *There We'll Meet Again*, 12 December 1914.
93   Sergeant Ernest Karganoff, French army, 1916, cited in Max Arthur, *Forgotten Voices of the Great War*. London: Ebury Press, 2002, p. 192.
94   Alfred Anderson, 5th Battalion, Black Watch, cited in Arthur, *Last Post*, p. 17.
95   W. Lockey, Nottingham and Derbyshire, The Sherwood Foresters, cited in Lyn MacDonald, *They Called It Passchendaele: The Story of the Third Battle of Ypres and of the Men who Fought in it*. London: Penguin, 1993 [1978], p. 115.
96   Jack Dorgan, 7th Battalion, Northumberland Fusiliers, cited in Arthur, *Forgotten Voices*, 1915, p. 91.
97   Cited in Jane Kimball, *Trench Art: An Illustrated History*. Davis, CA: Silverpenny Press, 2004, p. 38.
98   Alison Lurie, *The Language of Clothes*. London: Bloomsbury, 1992 [1981], p. 176.
99   Lyn Allyn and Clarence A. Bush, *Love from Chezeaux: WWI Memoirs of Clarence Bush*. Bloomington, IN: Author House, 2006, p. 50.
100 Ernst Jünger, *Storm of Steel*. London: Penguin, 2004, 17 October 1915.
101 Kimball, *Trench Art*, p. 41.
102 Harry Patch, June 1917, cited in Lyn MacDonald, *They Called it Passchendaele*, p. 125.

103 William Edward Finch, NCO with 2nd Battalion Worcestershire Regiment on the WF 1914, IWM 8280.

104 Niall Ferguson, *The Pity of War*. London: Allen Lane, 1998, p. 351.

105 Scott McFie, letter to father, cited in Lyn MacDonald, *1915: The Death of Innocence*, p. 396.

106 Bernard Britland, 14 February 1915, cited in Malcolm Brown, *The Imperial War Museum Book of the First World War*. London: Guild Publishing, 1991.

107 Mary Borden, *The Forbidden Zone: A Nurse's Impressions*. London: Hesperus Press, 2008 [1929], p. 39.

Chapter 5: Attitudes to the Body

1 Jonathan Miller, *The Body in Question*. London: Pimlico, 2000, p. 1.

2 Honoré Daumier, 1848.

3 Eugène Delacroix, *Liberty*, 1830.

4 William Ross Wallace, 1865.

5 David Wilson, IWM Q71311.

6 Raffael Schuster-Woldan, IWM PST 2684, 1918.

7 William Hatherell, IWM Art 5194, 1915.

8 Wilfred Owen, 'Hospital Barge at Cérisy'.

9 Owen, letter to mother, January 1917, cited in David Roberts, ed., *Minds at War: The Poetry and Experiences of the First World War*. Burgess Hill: Saxon, 1996, p. 312.

10 Helen Zenna Smith, ed., *Not So Quiet: Stepdaughters of War*. New York: The Feminist Press CUNY, 1978 [1930], p. 34.

11 Virginia Woolf, *Three Guineas*, 1938, cited in Nicoletta Gullace, *Women, War and Society 1914–1918*, www.gale.com/DigitalCollections.

12 Pat Barker, *Regeneration*. London: Penguin, 2008 [1991], pp. 107–8.

13 Ibid., p. 107.

14 Paul Fussell, ed., *The Ordeal of Alfred M Hale*. London: Leo Cooper, 1975, p. 77.

15 Ibid., p. 99.

16 Graham Seton, 'Biography of a Batman', *The English Review*, 1929.

17 The process of louse removal was known as 'chatting up', and could be done either with bare hands or lighted flames, sometimes with the help of naphthalene powder or paste.

18 Seton, 'Biography'.

19 Ibid.

20 Gaston Riou, *The Diary of a French Private: War Imprisonment, 1914–1915*. London: Allen and Unwin, 1916, IWM 14724, 1 July 1915.

21 Otto Braun, *The Diary of Otto Braun: With Selections of his Letters and Poems*. London: Heinemann, 1924, Graudenz, 30 September 1914.

22 J. C. Flügel, *The Psychology of Clothes*. London: Hogarth, 1950, p. 75.

23 Henry Williamson, *The Patriot's Progress*. Stroud: Sutton, 2004, p. 22.

24 Arthur Marwick, *The Deluge: British Society and the First World War*. London: Macmillan, 2006 [1965], p. 147.

25 Florence E. Booth, letter to *The Spectator*, 18 November 1916.

26 In 1912 Julius Fromm invented the 'cement dipping' technique, which resulted in less faults and a more even texture.

27 Shirley Green, *The Curious History of Contraception*. London: Ebury Press, 1971, p. 122.

28 James Woycke, *Birth Control In Germany, 1871–1933*. London: Routledge, 1998, p. 40.

29 Ibid., p. 51.

NOTES

30 Paul Fussell, *The Great War and Modern Memory*. Oxford: Oxford University Press, 2000 [1975], p. 271.
31 Braun, *Diary of Otto Braun*, Zehlendorf, 6 November 1917.
32 Cited in Clare Makepeace, 'Sex and the Trenches', *BBC History Magazine*, August 2011, vol. 12, no. 8, p. 48.
33 Lawrence James, *Warrior Race: A History of the British at War*. London: Abacus, 2001, p. 479.
34 Sergeant Alfred West, Monmouthshire Regiment, 1915, cited in Max Arthur, *Forgotten Voices of the Great War*. London: Ebury Press, 2002.
35 Robert Graves, *Goodbye To All That*. London: Penguin, 2011 [1929], The Red Lamp at Béthune, p. 125.
36 Private Sidney Albert Amatt, serving with 1/5th Battalion, London Regiment on the Western Front, 1916, IWM interview 9168.
37 Ellen Harriet, aka Charles Capon, *The Times*, 21 January 1918, cited in Moira Donald and Linda Hurcombe, *Representations of Gender*. London: Macmillan, 2000, p. 200.
38 C. Willett Cunnington, *Why Women Wear Clothes*. London: Faber and Faber, 1941, p. 203.
39 Charles Carrington (Edmonds), *A Subaltern's War: Being a Memoir of the Great War from the Point of View of a Romantic Young Man* ... London: Peter Davies, 1929, p. 188. The idea of 'sweet reasonableness' comes from Matthew Arnold, itself drawn from the New Testament, a translation perhaps of St Paul's 'gentleness' in 2 Corinthians.
40 Rumen Cholakov, 'Prisoners of War in Bulgaria during the First World War'. Cambridge University dissertation, 2012, p. 51.
41 'Enemy Images', in Karen Hagemann and Stefanie Schüler-Springorum, eds, *Home Front: The Military, War and Gender in Twentieth Century Germany*. Oxford: Berg, 2002, p. 143.
42 *Powers of Horror*, cited in Odile Krakovitch, 'Plus Ça Change', in Claire M. Tylee, ed., *Women, the First World War and Dramatic Imagination: International Essays, 1914–1999*. Lewiston, NY: Edwin Mellen Press, 2000, p. 232.
43 Hew Strachan, *The First World War: A New Illustrated History*. London: Simon and Schuster, 2003 p. 234.
44 Richard Aldington, 'Sunsets', in Brian Gardner, ed., *Up the Line to Death: The War Poets, 1914–1918*. London: Methuen, 1986 [1964], p. 109.
45 Edward Mousley, in Peter Englund, ed., *The Beauty and the Sorrow: An Intimate History of the First World War*. London: Profile, 2011, p. 269.
46 P. H. Pilditch, cited in Fussell, *The Great War and Modern Memory*, p. 241.
47 See Lindy Woodhead, *War Paint: Elizabeth Arden and Helena Rubenstein, their Lives, their Times, their Rivalry*. London: Virago, 2003.
48 Edmund Blunden, *Undertones of War*. London: Penguin, 2000.
49 Frederick Charles Higgins, NCO 4th Battalion Royal Fusiliers, Western Front 1915–17, IWM 9884.
50 Lieutenant Godfrey Buxton, 6th Battalion, Duke of Wellington's Regiment cited in Arthur, *Forgotten Voices*.
51 Mrs G. W. Gwatkin-Williams, *In the Hands of the Senoussi: The Story of the Nineteen Weeks Spent as Prisoners in the Libyan Desert by the Survivors of HMS 'Tara' and the Horse Transport 'Moorina', Compiled from the Diary of Captain R Gwatkin-Williams*. London: C. Arthur Pearson, 1916, pp. 74–5.
52 Ibid., p. 77.
53 Beth Daley, www.oucs.ox.uk/ww1.
54 'Body Damage: War Disability and Constructions of Masculinity in Weimar Germany', in Hagemann and Schüler-Springorum, eds, *Home Front*, p. 193.
55 Bright blue suits worn with a white shirt and red tie.

56 Neil Storey and Molly Housego, *Women in the First World War*. Princes Risborough: Shire, 2010, p. 61.

57 Catherine Horwood, 'Girls Who Arouse Dangerous Passions: Women and bathing 1900–39', *Women's History Review*, 2000, vol. 9, no. 4, p. 657.

58 Flügel, *The Psychology of Clothes*, p. 107.

59 Sarah Kennedy, *The Swimsuit*. London: Carlton Books, 2007.

60 David Kunzle, cited in Elizabeth Wilson, *Adorned in Dreams: Fashion and Modernity*. London: Virago, 1985, p. 99.

61 Ernie Williams, 6th Battalion Cheshire Regiment, IWM 25228.

Chapter 6: Entertaining Costume

1 Peter Jelavich, *Berlin Cabaret*. Cambridge, MA: Harvard University Press, 1993, p. 6.

2 Max Herrmann-Neisse, *Mein Weihnachtzwunsh furs Kabarett*, 1921, cited ibid., p. 106.

3 Susan Ingram and Katrina Sark, *Berliner Chic: A Locational History of Berlin Fashion*. Bristol: Intellect, 2011, p. 121.

4 Agnès Cardinal, 'Berta Lask's Befreiung: A Dramatic Experiment' in Claire M. Tylee, ed., *Women, the First World War and the Dramatic Imagination: International Essays, 1914–1999*. Lewiston, NY: Edwin Mellen Press, 2000, p. 122.

5 Musical comedy, written by Oscar Asche, record-breaking five-year run from 3 August 1916, His Majesty's Theatre.

6 Opened 19 April 1916, the first of three revues that ran until after the end of the War at the Alhambra Theatre.

7 Lewis A. Erenberg, *Steppin' Out: New York Nightlife and the Transformation of American Culture*. Chicago, IL: University of Chicago Press, 1984, p. 114.

8 http://philadancehistoryjournal.wordpress.com/tag/tango-teas/.

9 Kate Salter, 'Sonia Delaunay: a life of contrasts', *The Telegraph*, 31 July 2011.

10 Cited in Yvonne McEwan, *It's a Long Way to Tipperary: British and Irish Nurses in the Great War*. Dunfermline: Cualann Press, 2006, p. 26.

11 Odile Krakovitch, 'Plus Ça Change', in Claire M. Tylee, ed., *Women, the First World War and the Dramatic Imagination: International Essays, 1914–1999*. Lewiston, NY: Edwin Mellen Press, 2000, p. 60.

12 Holledge, cited in Tylee, ed., *Women*, p. 98.

13 IWM Q5327, Blangy, October 1917.

14 IWM Q5333, Chelers, May 1917.

15 IWM Q49578.

16 Apart from Sylvia Pankhurst and her supporters who were staunchly against the war.

17 Juliet Nicolson, *The Perfect Summer: Dancing into Shadow in 1911*. London: John Murray, 2006, p. 118.

18 Ibid., p. 119.

19 Mary E. Davis, *Ballets Russes Style: Diaghilev's Dancers and Paris Fashion*. London: Reaktion Books, 2010.

20 *Les Choses de Paul Poiret* series, 1911.

21 Anne Hollander, 'The Design is Always Right', in *New York Magazine*, 14 June 1974, p. 64.

22 Alison Adburgham, *Shops and Shopping: When and in What Manner the Well-Dressed Englishwoman Bought her Clothes*. London: Allen and Unwin, 1981 [1964], p. 249.

23 Hollander, 'The Design is Always Right', p. 65.

24 Mary E. Davis, *Classic Chic: Music, Fashion and Modernism*. Berkeley, CA: University of California Press, 2006, p. 165.

25 Cited in Davis, *Ballets Russes Style*, p. 197.

26 Davis, *Classic Chic*, p. 161.
27 Victoria Sherrow, *Encyclopedia of Hair: A Cultural History*. Westport CT: Greenwood Press, 2006, p. 49.

Chapter 7: Manufacture and the Home

1   Jane Cox, 1915, IWM 705.
2   Howard Watson Ambruster, *Treason's Peace*. Although the First World War reduced the German chemical output, over the next two decades it slowly regained ground so that at the beginning of the Second World War it was again a threat to Allied supplies.
3   www.woolworthmuseum.co.uk/1910s-ww1impact.htm.
4   Robert Graves, *Goodbye To All That*. London: Penguin, 2011 [1929] p. 156.
5   Edward M. Spiers, *A History of Chemical and Biological Warfare*. London: Reaktion Books, 2010, p. 40.
6   Lyn MacDonald, *1915: The Death of Innocence*. London: Headline, 1993, p. 232.
7   Sergeant Jack Dorgan, 7th Battalion Northumberland Fusiliers, cited in Max Arthur, *Forgotten Voices of the Great War*. London: Ebury Press, 2002, p. 82.
8   Graves, *Goodbye To All That*, 1914, p. 97.
9   Piete Kuhr, *There We'll Meet Again: A Young German Girl's Diary of the First World War*. London: Walter Wright, 1998 [1982 in German], 24 May 1915.
10 Graves, *Goodbye To All That*, p. 206.
11 Brian Resnick, 'What America Looked Like Collecting Peach Pits For World War One Gas Masks', 1 February 2012, www.theatlantic.com.
12 Lewis Baumer, 'An Uneasy Conscience', *Punch*, 8 March 1916.
13 Ibid., 'Economy in Dress: The New Smartness', *Punch*, 12 April 1916.
14 *The Great War*, 15 July 1916.
15 Alison Adburgham, *Shops and Shopping: When and in What Manner the Well-Dressed Englishwoman Bought her Clothes*. London: Allen and Unwin, 1981 [1964], p. 277.
16 Cited in Lindy Woodhead, *Shopping, Seduction and Mr Selfridge*. London: Profile Books, 2008, p. 136.
17 Susan Ingram and Katrina Sark, *Berliner Chic: A Locational History of Berlin Fashion*. Bristol: Intellect, 2011, p. 42.
18 Cited in Daniel Delis Hill, *As Seen in Vogue: A Century of American Fashion in Advertising*. Lubbock, TX: Texas Tech University Press, 2005, p. 27.
19 Hill, *As Seen in Vogue*, p. 30.
20 Ibid., p. 31.
21 Arthur Marwick, *The Deluge: British Society and the First World War*. London: Macmillan, 2006 [1965], p. 127.
22 Lindy Woodhead, *War Paint: Elizabeth Arden and Helena Rubenstein, their lives, their Times, their Rivalry*. London: Virago, 2003, p. 106.
23 *The Ealing Gazette*, 26 August 1914.
24 Adam Smith exemplifies the significance of this division of labour via the processes required in the manufacture of a pin in *An Inquiry into the Nature and Causes of the Wealth of Nations*, 1776.
25 http://www.costumes.org/history/100pages/nevamag.htm.
26 C. Willett Cunnington, *English Women's Clothing in the Present Century*. London: Faber and Faber, 1952, p. 141.
27 Kuhr, *There We'll Meet Again*, 3 August 1914.
28 Niall Ferguson, *The Pity of War*. London: Allen Lane, 1998, p. 350.

29 N. Robertson, 'A Woman's Prayer', in Susan M. Strawn, *Knitting America: A Glorious Heritage of Warm Socks to High Art*. Minneapolis: Motorbooks International, 2007, p. 91.
30 Strawn, *Knitting America*, pp. 92–6.
31 Ibid.
32 Cunnington, *English Women's Clothing*, p. 138.
33 Evangeline Booth and Grace Livingston Hill, *The War Romance of the Salvation Army*. London: J. B. Lippincott, 1919, p. 13.
34 *The Great War*, 15 July 1916, p. 555.
35 Helen Bosanquet, 'The Old Woman's War-Work', in Nosheen Khan, *Women's Poetry of the First World War*. Lexington, KY: University of Kentucky, 1988.
36 *Petit Sous, Que Deviendrez-Vous?* (What will become of you, little pennies?) Sim Bangley, IWM Art 12879.
37 *Sammelt: Frauenhaar!* (Collect women's hair!), Hausdruckerie Drägerwerk, IWM Art 12933.
38 Elizabeth Owen, 1914, in Arthur, *Forgotten Voices*.
39 Jennie Lee, *My Life with Nye*. London: Cape, 1980, p. 28.
40 Kuhr, *There We'll Meet Again*, 25 September 1914.
41 Barbara Sleigh, *The Smell of Privet*. London: Hutchinson, 1971, p. 111.
42 IWM EPH 10385.
43 Lyn Ferguson, *The Pity of War*, p. 229.
44 IWM EPH 3801.
45 IWM 30172.
46 MacDonald, *1915: The Death of Innocence*, p. 6.
47 Ibid., p. 7.
48 Lettice Miller, IWM 14241.
49 Anna Eisenmenger, cited in Hew Strachan, *The First World War: A New Illustrated History*. London: Simon and Schuster, 2003 p. 329.

Chapter 8: Death, Marriage and Identity

1 Lady Duff Gordon, *Discretions and Indiscretions*, cited in Lou Taylor, *Mourning Dress: A Costume and Social History*. London: Routledge, 2009 [1983], p. 266.
2 Piete Kuhr, *There We'll Meet Again: A Young German Girl's Diary of the First World War*. London: Walter Wright, 1998 [1982 in German], 24 December 1914.
3 Edna Woolman Chase and Ilka Chase, *Always in Vogue*. New York: Gollancz, 1954, p. 100.
4 Taylor, *Mourning Dress*, p. 269.
5 Valerie Steele, *Paris Fashion: A Cultural History*. Oxford: Berg, 1998, p. 30.
6 Taylor, *Mourning Dress*, pp. 270–1.
7 Anne Hollander, *Seeing Through Clothes*. Berkeley, CA: University of California Press, 1993, p. 382.
8 Taylor, *Mourning Dress*, p. 272.
9 Vera Brittain, 13 January 1916, in Joyce Marlow, ed., *The Virago Book of Women and the Great War*. London: Virago, 2005 [1998], pp. 195–6.
10 Ibid.
11 Taylor, *Mourning Dress*, p. 185.
12 Amy Elizabeth May, IWM 684.
13 Ibid., p. 16.
14 IWM NTB 224-1.
15 http://www.westernfrontassociation.com.
16 Henry Williamson, *The Patriot's Progress*. Stroud: Sutton, 2004 [1930], p.175.
17 www.abc.net.au/news/specials/fromelles-fallen/.

NOTES

Chapter 9: O Brave New World

1   Ruth Cowen, ed., *War Diaries, A Nurse at the Front: The First World War Diaries of Sister Edith Appleton.* London: IWM and Simon and Schuster, 2012, p. 263.

2   Philipp Witkop, *German Students' War Letters.* Philadelphia, PA: Pine Street Books, 2013, p. 218.

3   Charles Ward, Middlesex Regiment, Purfleet 1920, IWM 12026.

4   Ibid.

5   Corporal T. Whittaker, King's Own Royal Lancaster Regiment, www. nyt.co.uk/warletter.

6   IWM 18834.

7   *The Field Service Notebook 1914,* '38. Clothing', p. 181.

8   The fashion for wearing uniform in the 1960s was decried by some, and individuals were threatened in letters to the *Daily Telegraph* with the 1894 Act.

9   Susan R. Grayzel, *Women's Identities at War: Gender, Motherhood and Politics in Britain and France during the First World War.* Chapel Hill, NC: University of North Carolina Press, 1999, p. 224.

10   Reverend Andrew Clark, in Steve Humphries and Richard van Emden, *All Quiet on the Home Front: An Oral History of Life in Britain during the First World War.* London: Headline, 2004, p. 302.

11   Ian Beckett, *Home Front, 1914–1918: How Britain Survived the Great War.* The National Archives, 2006.

12   David Mitchell, *Women on the Warpath: The Story of the Women of the First World War.* London: Jonathan Cape, 1966, p. 224.

13   C. Willett Cunnington, *English Women's Clothing in the Present Century.* London: Faber and Faber, 1952, p. 150.

14   Anne Hollander, *Seeing Through Clothes.* Berkeley, CA: University of California Press, 1993, p. 8.

15   See Marwick (*War and Social Change in the Twentieth Century: A Comparative Study of Britain, France, Germany, Russia and the United States*) and women's 'liberation' as opposed to stasis in Sylvia Walby, *Patriarchy at Work,* p. 156, and for a breakdown of different viewpoints, Angela Woollacott, *On Her Their Lives Depend: Munitions Workers in the Great War.*

16   Daniel D. Hill, *As Seen in Vogue: A Century of American Fashion in Advertising.* Lubbock, TX: Texas Tech University Press, 2005, p. 33.

17   *The Daily Sketch,* 21 October 1924, cited in Aileen Ribiero, *Dress and Morality.* London: Batsford, 1986, p. 24.

18   Lindy Woodhead, *Shopping, Seduction and Mr Selfridge.* London: Profile Books, 2008, p. 162.

19   Victoria Sherrow, *Encyclopedia of Hair: A Cultural History.* Westport CT: Greenwood Press, 2006, p. 64.

20   James Laver p. 110, in Elizabeth Wilson, *Adorned in Dreams: Fashion and Modernity.* London: Virago, 1985, p. 103.

21   Laurence Senelick, 'Cabaret Performance' in *Europe, 1920–1940.* Volume 1, Baltimore, MD: Johns Hopkins University Press, 1993, p. 25.

22   Mila Ganeva, *Women in Weimar Fashion: Discourses and Displays in German Culture, 1918–33.* New York: Camden House, 2008, p. 40.

23   Paul Connerton, *The Spirit of Mourning: History, Memory and the Body.* Cambridge University Press, 2011, p. 28.

24   Mary E. Davis, *Classic Chic: Music, Fashion and Modernism.* Berkeley, CA: University of California Press, 2006, p. 163.

25 Catherine Horwood, 'Girls Who Arouse Dangerous Passions: Women and bathing 1900–39', *Women's History Review*, 2000, vol. 9, no. 4, p. 658.
26 *The Lady*, 'Pomeroy Summer Treatments', 22 August 1918.
27 Jennifer Craik, *Uniforms Exposed: From Conformity to Transgression*. Oxford: Berg, 2005, p. 65.

Conclusion

1 Claude Choules 1901–2011, *The Last of the Last*. Edinburgh: Mainstream, 2010, p. 39.
2 Ibid., p. 90.

GLOSSARY

APMMC	Almeric Paget Military Massage Corps
BASC	British Army Service Corps
Central Powers	Germany and Austro-Hungary (after the Triple Alliance of 1882 which had included Italy), and joined during the First World War by the Ottoman Empire/Turkey and Bulgaria
Entente Cordiale	agreement between France and Britain, 1904, principally over Morocco and Egypt
FANYs	First Aid Nursing Yeomanry
IWM	Imperial War Museum
NCO	non-commissioned officer
Neutrals	the Netherlands, Switzerland, Spain, Denmark, Sweden and Norway
POW	prisoner of war
QAIMNS	Queen Alexandra's Imperial Military Nursing Service
TNT	trinitrotoluene, used as an explosive agent and a by-product of dye manufacture
Triple Entente	between Russia, France and Britain, 1907, and joined during the First World War by Romania, Portugal, Greece, Japan, and Italy, and later by the United States of America in 1917
VAD	Voluntary Aid Detachments
WAAC	Women's Army Auxiliary Corps
WF	Western Front
WVR	Women's Voluntary Reserve

BIBLIOGRAPHY

Adburgham, Alison. *Shops and Shopping: Where and in What Manner the Well-dressed Englishwomen Bought Her Clothes*. London: Allen and Unwin, 1981 [1964]

Adie, Kate. *Corsets to Camouflage: Women and War*. London: Hodder and Stoughton, 2003

Allen, Dan. *Ladies in Uniform*. Soldiers of the Queen 118

Allyn, Lyn and Bush, Clarence A. *Love from Chezeaux: WWI Memoirs of Clarence Bush*. Bloomington, IN: Author House, 2006

Ambruster, Howard Watson. *Treason's Peace: German Dyes and American Dupes*. New York: Beechhurst Press, 1947

Anderson, Gregory, ed. *White Blouse Revolution: Female Office Workers since 1870*. Manchester: Manchester University Press, 1988

Anderson, Perry. 'Modernity and Revolution', in *New Left Review*, no. 144, 1984

Angeloglou, Maggie. *A History of Makeup*. Worthing: Littlehampton Book Services, 1970

Arthur, Max. *Forgotten Voices of the Great War*. London: Ebury Press, 2002

—— *Last Post*. London: Weidenfeld & Nicolson, 2005

Arthur, Terri. *Fatal Decision: Edith Cavell, World War One Nurse*. Milpitas: Beagle Books, 2011

Bajohr, Stefan. *Die Hälfte der Fabrik. Geschichte der Frauenarbeit in Deutschland, 1914–1945, [Half of the Factory: The History of Women's Employment in Germany, 1914–1945]*. Marburg: Verlay Arbeiterbewegung und Gesellschaftswissenschaft, 1979

Bancroft, Alison. *Fashion and Psychoanalysis: Styling the Self*. London: I.B.Tauris, 2012

Barker, Pat. *Regeneration*. London: Penguin, 2008 [1991]

Barnes, Annie, Harding, Kate and Gibbs, Caroline. *Tough Annie: From Suffragette to Stepney Councillor*. London: Stepney Books Publications, 1980

Barthes, Roland. *The Fashion System*. Berkeley, CA: University of California Press, 1992

Batchelor, David. *Chromophobia*. London: Reaktion Books, 2011

Battersby, M. *Art Deco Fashion: French Designers, 1908–25*. London: Academy Editions, 1984

Beaulieu, Denyse. *The Perfume Lover: A Personal History of Scent*. London: HarperCollins, 2012

Beckett, Ian. *Home Front, 1914–1918: How Britain Survived the Great War*. The National Archives, 2006

Beer, John J. *The Emergence of the German Dye Industry*. n.p. Ayer Co., 1981 [1959]

Bell, Quentin. *On Human Finery*. London: Hogarth Press, 1976

Benton, Tim, Benton, Charlotte and Wood, Ghislaine. *Art Deco: 1910–39*. London: V&A Publications, 2003

Bertin, Célia. *Paris à la Mode: A Voyage of Discovery*. London: Victor Gollanz, 1956

Bishop, Alan and Bostridge, Mark, eds. *Letters from a Lost Generation: First World War Letters of Vera Brittain and Four Friends*. London: Abacus, 1998

Blau, Herbert. *Nothing In Itself: Complexions of Fashion*. Bloomington, IN: Indiana University Press, 1999

Blunden, Edmund. *Undertones of War*. London: Penguin, 2000

Booth, Evangeline and Livingston Hill, Grace. *The War Romance of the Salvation Army*, London: J. B. Lippincott, 1919

Borden, Mary. *The Forbidden Zone: A Nurse's Impressions*. London: Hesperus Press, 2008 [1929]

Bowley, A. L. *Some Economic Consequences of the Great War*. London: Thornton Butterworth, 1930

Braun, Otto, Winter, Ella, trans., Browne, Stella trans. poetry. *The Diary of Otto Braun: With Selections of his Letters and Poems*. London: Heinemann, 1924

Brayley, Martin and Ingram, Richard. *World War II, British Women's Uniforms*. London: Windrow and Greene, 1995

Brittain, Vera. *Testament of Youth*. London: Virago, 1988 [1933]

Broadberry, Stephen and Harrison, Mark, eds. *The Economics of World War One*. Cambridge: Cambridge University Press, 2005

Broadberry, Stephen and Howlett, Peter. 'The United Kingdom during World War One: Business as Usual', in S. Broadberry and M. Harrison, eds. *The Economics of World War I*. Cambridge: Cambridge University Press, 2005, pp. 206–34

Brown, Malcolm. *The Imperial War Museum Book of the First World War*. London: Guild Publishing, 1991

Buchan, John. *Greenmantle*. Oxford: Oxford World Classics, 1993 [1916]

Buckle, Henry. *A Tommy's Sketchbook: Writings and Drawings from the Trenches*. Stroud: The History Press, 2012

Buckley, Cheryl. 'De-Humanized Females and Amazonians: British wartime fashion and its representation in *Home Chat*, 1914–1918', in *Gender and History*, Oxford: Blackwell, November 2002, vol. 14, no. 3, pp. 516–36

Buckley, Cheryl and Hilary Fawcett. *Fashioning the Feminine: Representation and Women's Fashion from the Fin de Siècle to the Present*. London: I.B.Tauris, 2001

Bum, Stella, ed. *Everyday Fashions of the Twenties: As Pictured in Sears and other Catalogues*. New York: Dover Publications, 1981

Buxbaum, Gerda, ed. *Icons of Fashion, the 20th Century*. London: Prestel, 2000

Cardinal, Agnès. 'Berta Lask's Die Befreiung: A dramatic experiment', in Claire M. Tylee, ed. *Women, the First World War and the Dramatic Imagination: International Essays, 1914–1999*. Lewiston, NY: Edwin Mellen Press, 2000

Carrington, Charles (Charles Edmonds), *A Subaltern's War: Being a Memoir of the Great War from the Point of View of a Romantic Young Man* ... London: Peter Davies, 1929

Cassin-Scott, Jack. *Women at War: 1939–45*. New York: Osprey, 1980

Cate, Clifton J. and Cate, Charles Cameron. *Notes: A Soldier's Memoir of World War One*. Victoria, BC: Trafford, 2005

Chambers, Steve. *Uniforms and Equipment of the British Army in World War One: A Study in Period Photographs*. Atglen, PA: Schiffer Books, 2004

Chase, Edna Woolman and Chase, Ilka. *Always in Vogue*. New York: Gollancz, 1954

Cholakov, Rumen. 'Prisoners of War in Bulgaria during the First World War'. Cambridge University dissertation, 2012

Chopin, Kate. *The Awakening and Selected Stories*. Harmondsworth: Penguin, 1984 [1899]

Choules, Claude. *The Last of the Last*. Edinburgh: Mainstream, 2010

Van Cleave, Kendra. 'Fashion', in James Ciment and Thadeus Russell, *The Home Front Encyclopedia: United States, Britain and Canada in World War I and II*. Santa Barbara: ABC-CLIO, 2006

Collins, Amy Fine. 'Toujours Couture', in *Vanity Fair*, September 2009

Connerton, Paul. *The Spirit of Mourning: History, Memory and the Body*. Cambridge: Cambridge University Press, 2011

Cowen, Ruth, ed. *War Diaries, A Nurse at the Front: The First World War Diaries of Sister Edith Appleton*. London: IWM and Simon and Schuster, 2012

Cowman, Keith and Jackson, Louisa Ainsley. *Women and Work Culture, 1850–1950*. Aldershot: Ashgate, 2005

Cox, Caroline. *Good Hair Days: A History of British Hairdressing*. London: Quartet, 1999

Craik, Jennifer. *Uniforms Exposed: From Conformity to Transgression*. Oxford: Berg, 2005

Cumming, Valerie. *Understanding Fashion History*. London: Batsford, 2011

Cunnington, C. Willett. *Why Women Wear Clothes*. London: Faber and Faber, 1941

—— *English Women's Clothing in the Present Century*. London: Faber and Faber, 1952

Damhorst, Mary Lynn, Miller, Kimberly A. and Michelman, Susan O. *The Meanings of Dress*. New York: Fairchild Publications, 1999

Damousi, Joy. *Gender and War: Australians at War in the Twentieth Century*. Cambridge: Cambridge University Press, 1995

Davis, Fred. *Fashion, Culture and Identity*. Chicago, IL: University of Chicago Press, 1994

Davis, Mary E. *Classic Chic: Music, Fashion and Modernism*. Berkeley, CA: University of California Press, 2006

—— *Ballets Russes Style: Diaghilev's Dancers and Paris Fashion*. London: Reaktion Books, 2010

De Courtais, Georgine. *Women's Hats, Headdresses, Hairstyles*. New York: Dover Publications, 2006 [1973]

de la Haye, Amy. *Land Girls: Cinderellas of the Soil*. Museum and Art Gallery of Brighton catalogue, 2009/10

De Watteville, H. 'The Royal Army Clothing Department', in *RUSI Journal*, 1932, vol. 77, issue 507

Dobbs, S. P. *The Clothing Workers of Great Britain*. London: Routledge, 2005 [1928]

Donald, Moira and Hurcombe, Linda. *Representations of Gender*. London: Macmillan, 2000.

Doyle, Peter. *British Postcards of the First World War*. Princes Risborough: Shire Publications, 2010

Edmonds, James Edward. *Military Operations, France and Belgium 1914*, Volume 1. London: HMSO, 1925

Eisenstein, Hester. *Gender Shock*. London: Allen and Unwin, 1991

Ellsworth-Jones, Will. *We Will Not Fight: The Untold Story of World War One's Conscientious Objectors*. London: Aurum Press, 2008

Englund, Peter. *The Beauty and the Sorrow: An Intimate History of the First World War*. London: Profile, 2011

Enloe, Cynthia H. *Maneuvers: The International Politics of Militarizing Women's Lives*. Berkeley, CA: University of California Press, 2000

Entwistle, Joanne. *The Fashioned Body: Fashion, Dress and Modern Social Theory*. Cambridge: Polity Press, 2000

Epstein, Diana. *The Button Book*. London: Running Press, 1996

Erenberg, Lewis A. *Steppin' Out: New York Nightlife and the Transformation of American Culture*. Chicago, IL: University of Chicago Press, 1984

Ewing, Elizabeth. *Women in Uniform through the Centuries*, London: Batsford, 1975

Faulks, Sebastian. *Birdsong*. London: Vintage, 1994 [1993]

Ferguson, Niall. *The Pity of War*. London: Allen Lane, 1998

Ferry, John William. *A History of the Department Store*. New York: Macmillan, 1960

Finn, Bernard and Hacker, Barton C. *Materializing the Military*. Washington DC: Smithsonian Institution, 2005

Fitzgerald, F. Scott. *Tender is the Night*. Harmondsworth: Penguin, 1997 [1934]

Flanner, Janet. *Paris Was Yesterday, 1925–39*. New York: Penguin, 1979

Flügel, J. C. *The Psychology of Clothes*. London: Hogarth, 1950

Flusser, Alan. *Dressing the Man*. London: HarperCollins, 2003

Fowler, W. W. *Nazi Regalia*. Bel Air, CA: Chartwell Books, 1998

Fraser, Grace Lovat. *Textiles by Britain*. London: Allen and Unwin, 1948

Fussell, Paul. *The Great War and Modern Memory*. Oxford: Oxford University Press, 2000 [1975]

—— *Uniforms: Why we Are What we Wear.* New York: Mariner Books, 2002

Fussell, Paul, ed. *The Ordeal of Alfred M Hale.* London: Leo Cooper, 1975

Ganeva, Mila. *Women in Weimar Fashion: Discourses and Displays in German Culture, 1918–33.* New York: Camden House, 2008

Gardner, Brian, ed. *Up the Line to Death: The War Poets, 1914–1918.* London: Methuen, 1986 [1964]

Gest, Kevin L. *Chivalry: The Origins and History of the Orders of Knighthood.* Hersham: Ian Allen, 2010

Gilbert, Pam and Taylor, Sandra. *Fashioning the Feminine: Girls, Popular Culture and Schooling.* London: Allen and Unwin, 1991

Gilbert, Sandra. 'Soldier's Heart', in *Signs 8*, no. 3, Spring 1983

Gilbert, Sandra M. and Gubar, Susan. 'No Man's Land, the Place of the Woman Writer in the Twentieth Century', in *Sexchanges*, Volume 2. New Haven, CT: Yale University Press, 1989

Gill, Thomas. *Life On All Fronts.* Cambridge: Cambridge University Press, 1989

Graves, Robert. *Goodbye To All That.* London: Penguin, 2011 [1929]

Grayzel, Susan R. *Women's Identities at War: Gender, Motherhood and Politics in Britain and France during the First World War.* Chapel Hill, NC: University of North Carolina Press, 1999

—— *Women and the First World War.* Harlow: Longman, 2002

Green, Shirley. *The Curious History of Contraception.* London: Ebury Press, 1971

Gullace, Nicoletta F. 'Female Patriotism in the Great War', in *Women, War and Society 1914–1918*, www.gale.com/DigitalCollections

—— 'Sexual Violence and Family Honor: British propaganda and international law during the First World War', in *The American Historical Review*, June 1997

Gwatkin-Williams, Mrs G. W. *In the Hands of the Senoussi: The Story of the Nineteen Weeks Spent as Prisoners in the Libyan Desert by the Survivors of HMS 'Tara' and the Horse Transport 'Moorina', Compiled from the Diary of Captain R Gwatkin-Williams.* London: C. Arthur Pearson, 1916

Hagemann, Karen and Schüler-Springorum, Stefanie, eds. *Home Front: The Military, War and Gender in Twentieth Century Germany.* Oxford: Berg, 2002

Harris, Carol. *Women at War: 1939–45.* Stroud: The History Press, 2002

Harvey, John. *Men in Black.* London: Reaktion Books, 1995

Hatt, Christine. *The First World War, 1914–18.* London: Evans Brothers, 2000

Hay, Margaret Jean. 'The Importance of Clothing and Struggles over Identity in Colonial Western Kenya', in *Fashioning Africa: Power and the Politics of Dress*, ed. Jean Allman, Bloomington, IN: Indiana University Press, 2004

Heyman, Neil M. *World War One.* Westport, CT: Greenwood Press, 1997

Hibberd, Dominic, ed. *Poetry of the First World War.* London: Macmillan Education, 1987 [1981]

Higonnet, Margaret R., Jenson, Jane, Michel, Sonya and Collins Weitz, Margaret, eds. *Behind the Lines: Gender and the Two World Wars.* New Haven, CT: Yale University Press, 1987

Hill, Daniel Delis. *As Seen in Vogue: A Century of American Fashion in Advertising.* Lubbock, TX: Texas Tech University Press, 2005

His, Wilhelm, Blech, Gustavus M. and Kean, Jefferson R., trans. *A German Doctor at the Front.* Washington DC: The National Service Publishing Company, 1933

Holland, Samantha. *Alternative Femininities: Body, Age and Identity.* Oxford: Berg, 2004

Hollander, Anne. *Seeing Through Clothes.* Berkeley, CA: University of California Press, 1993

Holledge, Julie. *Innocent Flowers.* London: Virago, 1981

Holmes, Richard. *Tommy: The British Soldier on the Western Front 1914–1918.* London: Harper Perennial, 2004

Honig, Bonnie. *Feminist Interpretations of Hannah Arendt.* University Park, PA: Pennsylvania State University Press, 1995

Hope, Christine. 'Caucasian Female Body Hair and American Culture', in *Journal of American Culture*, 2004, vol. 5, issue 1

Hopkins, Sylvia. *Clothing for the Female Soldier*. London: Uniform Department of the National Army Museum, *c.*1990s

Horwood, C. 'Girls Who Arouse Dangerous Passions: Women and bathing 1900–39', in *Women's History Review*, 2000, vol. 9, no. 4, pp. 653–73

Humphries, Steve and Van Emden, Richard. *All Quiet on the Home Front: An Oral History of Life in Britain during the First World War*. London: Headline, 2004

Ingram, Susan and Katrina Sark. *Berliner Chic: A Locational History of Berlin Fashion*. Bristol: Intellect, 2011

James, Lawrence. *Warrior Race: A History of the British at War*. London: Abacus, 2001

Jelavich, Peter. *Berlin Cabaret*. Cambridge, MA: Harvard University Press, 1993

Jünger, Ernst, Hofmann, Michael, trans. *Storm of Steel*. London: Penguin, 2004 [1930 in German]

Keegan, John. *World Armies*. London: Macmillan, 1983 [1979]

Kennedy, Sarah. *The Swimsuit*. London: Carlton Books, 2007

Khan, Nosheen. *Women's Poetry of the First World War*. Lexington, KY: University of Kentucky, 1988

Kimball, Jane A. *Trench Art: An Illustrated History*. Davis, CA: Silverpenny Press, 2004

Kramer, Ann. *Women and War, WWI*. London: Franklin Watts, 2004

Kraus, Jürgen. *The German Army in the First World War: Uniforms and Equipment, 1914–1918*. Vienna: Militaria Verlag, 2006

Kraus, Jürgen and Schlicht, Adolf. *The German Reichswehr: Uniforms and Equipment of the German Army, 1919–1932*. Vienna: Militaria Verlag, 2006

Kuhr, Piete. Wright, Walter, trans. *There We'll Meet Again: A Young German Girl's Diary of the First World War*. London: Walter Wright, 1998 [1982 in German]

Lansdell, Avril. *Everyday Fashions of the Twentieth Century*. Princes Risborough: Shire Publications, 1999

Laver, James. *Taste and Fashion*. London: Harrap, 1948

—— *A Concise History of Costume*. London: Thames and Hudson, 1969

Lee, Jennie. *My Life with Nye*. London: Cape, 1980

Van Leeuwen, Mary Stewart. *A Sword Between the Sexes? C. S. Lewis and the Gender Debates*. Ada MI: Brazos Press, 2010

Lurie, Alison. *The Language of Clothes*. London: Bloomsbury, 1992 [1981]

MacDonald, Lyn. *Somme*. London: Penguin, 1983

—— *1914: The Days of Hope*. Harmondsworth: Penguin, 1987

—— *1915: The Death of Innocence*. London: Headline, 1993

—— *The Roses of No Man's Land*, Harmondsworth: Penguin, 1993 [1980]

—— *They Called It Passchendaele: The Story of the Third Battle of Ypres and of the Men who Fought in it*. London: Penguin, 1993 [1978]

MacDonald, Robin. 'White Feather Feminism: The recalcitrant progeny of radical suffragist and conservative pro-war Britain', Fort Myers, FL: Florida Gulf Coast University, 1998 http://itech.fgcu.edu/&/issue1/feather.htm

MacKenzie, Althea. *Shoes and Slippers: One of the World's Leading Collections of Costume and Accessory of the 18th and 19th Centuries*. Swindon: National Trust Books, 2006

Maitland, Sara. *Vesta Tilley*. London: Virago, 1986

Makepeace, Clare, 'Sex and the Trenches', *BBC History Magazine*, August 2011, vol. 12, no. 8, pp. 48–9

Marcus, Jane. 'The Asylums of Antaeus: Women, war and madness', in *The Difference Within*. Elizabeth A. Meese and Alice A. Parker, eds. Amsterdam: John Benjamins, 1989

Marlow, Joyce, ed. *The Virago Book of Women and the Great War*. London: Virago, 2005 [1998]

Martin, Sara. *Women and World War One*. www.firstworldwar.com

Marwick, Arthur. *War and Social Change in the Twentieth Century: A Comparative Study of Britain, France, Germany, Russia and the United States*. New York: St Martin's Press, 1974

—— *The Great War – and Modern Memory*. Oxford: Oxford University Press, 1975

—— *Women at War, 1914–1918*. London: Fontana for the Imperial War Museum, 1977

—— *The Deluge: British Society and the First World War*. London: Macmillan, 2006 [1965]

Marwick, Arthur, ed. *Total War and Historical Change: Europe, 1914–55*. Milton Keynes and Philadelphia, PA: Open University Press, 2001

McCoole, Sinéad. *No Ordinary Women: Irish Female Activists in the Revolutionary Years, 1900–1923*. Dublin: The O'Brien Press, 2003

McEwen, Yvonne. *It's a Long Way to Tipperary: British and Irish Nurses in the Great War*. Dunfermline: Cualann Press, 2006

McGreal Stephen. *The War on Hospital Ships, 1914–1918*. Barnsley: Pen and Sword Maritime, 2008

McKay, Malcolm. *Forgotten Voices*. London: Oberon, 2007

McLaven, Angus. *A History of Contraception: From Antiquity to the Present Day*. Oxford: Blackwell, 1990

Miller, Jonathan. *The Body in Question*. London: Pimlico 2000

Miller, Louise. *A Fine Brother: The Life of Captain Flora Sandes*. London: Alma Books, 2012

Milward, A. S. *The Economic Effects of the Two World Wars on Britain*. 2nd edn. London: Macmillan, 1984

Mindel, Adrian, ed. *Condoms*. London: BMJ Books, 2000

Mitchell, David John. *Monstrous Regiment*. London: Macmillan, 1965

—— *Women on the Warpath: The Story of the Women of the First World War*. London: Jonathan Cape, 1966

Mollo, John. *Military Fashion: A Comparative History of the Uniforms of the Great Armies of the Seventeenth Century to the First World War*. London: Barrie and Jenkins, 1972

Motion, Andrew. 'Anthem on Doomed Youth', in *Saturday Guardian*, 13 November 2011

Munson, James, ed. *Echoes of the Great War: The Diary of Rev Andrew Clark, 1914–19*. Oxford: Oxford University Press, 1985

Myers, Walter Dean and Miles, Bill. *The Harlem Hellfighters*, London: HarperCollins, 2006

Newton, Stella Mary. *Health, Art and Reason: Dress Reformers of the 19th Century*. London: John Murray, 1974

Nicolson, Juliet. *The Perfect Summer: Dancing into Shadow in 1911*. London: John Murray, 2006

Nystrom, Paul Henry. *Economics of Fashion*. New York: Ronald Press, 1928

Ollerenshaw, Philip. 'Textile business in Europe during the First World War, 1914–1918'. *Business History*, January 1999, vol. 41, issue 1, pp. 63–7

Osborne, Frances. *The Bolter: Idina Sackville – The Woman who Scandalised 1920s Society and Became White Mischief's Infamous Seductress*. London: Virago, 2008

Peck, Charles E. *Allen Peck's WWI Letters Home, 1917–1919: US Army WWI Pilot Assigned to France*. New York, NY: iUniverse, 2005

Pedersen, Stephanie. *BRA: A Thousand Years of Style, Support and Seduction*. Newton Abbot: David and Charles, 2004

Pfanner, Toni. 'Military Uniforms and the Law of War', *IRRC*, March 2004, vol. 86, no. 853, pp. 93–124

Popham, Hugh. *FANY: The Story of the Women's Transport Service, 1907–84*. London: Secker and Warburg, 1984

Poplin, Irene Schuessler. 'Nursing uniforms: Romantic idea, functional allure or instrument of social change?', in *Nursing History Review 2*, 1994, pp. 153–67

Powell, Anne. *Women in the War Zone: Hospital Service in the First World War*. Stroud: The History Press, 2001

—— *Women Doctors and Nurses on the Western and Eastern Fronts During the First World War*, http://www.millicentsutherlandambulance.com

Probert, Christina. *Brides in Vogue since 1910*. London: Thames and Hudson, 1984

Reilly, Catherine W., ed. *Scars Upon My Heart: Women's Poetry and Verse of the First World War*. London: Virago, 1981

Remarque, Erich Maria, trans. Brian Murdoch. *All Quiet on the Western Front*. London: Vintage, 1996 [1929]

Ribiero, Aileen. *Dress and Morality*. London: Batsford, 1986

Riello, Giorgio. *Shoes: A History from Sandals to Sneakers*. New York: Macmillan, 2011

Riou, Gaston. Paul, Eden and Cedar, trans. *The Diary of a French Private: War Imprisonment, 1914–1915*. London: Allen and Unwin, 1916, IWM 14724

Roberts, David, ed. *Minds at War: The Poetry and Experience of the First World War*. Burgess Hill: Saxon, 1996

Robinson, Jane. *Bluestockings: The Remarkable Story of the First Women to Fight for an Education*. London: Profile, 2009

Roderigues, Justina. *The Debate Over Women's Clothes: Rational or Lady-like Dress*. www.loyno.edu/-history/journal/1989-0/roderigues.htm

Salmonson, Jessica Amanda. *The Encyclopedia of Amazons: Women Warriors from Antiquity to the Modern Era*. London: Paragon House, 1991

Sassoon, Siegfried. *Memoirs of an Infantry Officer*. London: Faber and Faber, 1989 [1930]

Senelick, Laurence. 'Cabaret Performance', in *Europe, 1920–1940*, Volume 1. Baltimore, MD: Johns Hopkins University Press, 1993

Seton, Graham. 'Biography of a Batman'. *The English Review*, 1929

Sherrow, Victoria. *Encyclopedia of Hair: A Cultural History*. Westport CT: Greenwood Press, 2006

Shipman, Pat. *Femme Fatale: Love, Lies and the Unknown Life of Mata Hari*. New York: Harper Collins, 2007

Sleigh, Barbara. *The Smell of Privet*. London: Hutchinson, 1971

Smith, Helen Zenna, ed. *Not So Quiet: Stepdaughters of War*. New York: The Feminist Press CUNY, 1978 [1930]

Spiers, Edward M. *A History of Chemical and Biological Weapons*. London: Reaktion Books, 2010

Steele, Valerie. *Paris Fashion: A Cultural History*. Oxford: Berg, 1998

—— *The Corset: A Cultural History*. New Haven, CT: Yale University Press, 2003

Stewart, Alexander. *The Experiences of a Very Unimportant Officer*. London: Hodder, 2009.

Stewart, Susan. *On Longing: Narratives of the Miniature, the Gigantic, the Souvenir, the Collection*. Durham, NC: Duke University Press, 1993

Stoff, Laurie S. *They Fought for the Motherland: Russia's Women Soldiers in WWI and the Revolution*. Lawrence, KS: University of Kansas Press, 2006

Stone, Norman. *World War One: A Short History*. New York: Basic Books, 2009

Storey, Neil and Housego, Molly. *Women in the First World War*. Princes Risborough: Shire, 2010

Strachan, Hew. *The First World War: A New Illustrated History*. London: Simon and Schuster, 2003

—— *Financing the First World War*. Oxford: Oxford University Press, 2004

Strawn, Susan M. *Knitting America: A Glorious Heritage from Warm Socks to High Art*. Minneapolis, MN: Motorbooks International, 2007

Takeda, S. and Spilker, K. *Fashioning Fashion: European Dress, 1700–1915*. London: Prestel, 2010

Tardi, Jacques and Verney, Jean-Pierre. *Goddamn This War*. Seattle, WA: Fantagraphics, 2013

Taylor, A. J. P. *The First World War: An Illustrated History*. London: Penguin, 1966 [1963]

Taylor, Lou. *Mourning Dress: A Costume and Social History*. London: Routledge, 2009 [1983]

Thom, Deborah. *Nice Girls and Rude Girls: Women Workers in World War One*. London: I.B.Tauris, 1998

Tuchman, Barbara W. *The Guns of August: The Outstanding Account of the Outbreak of the First World War*. London: Constable and Robinson, 2000 [1962]

Tylee, Claire M. *The Great War and Women's Consciousness*. Iowa City: University of Iowa Press, 1990

—— ed. *Women, The First World War and the Dramatic Imagination: International Essays, 1914–1999*. Lewiston, NY: Edwin Mellen Press, 2000

Tyrer, Zinna Nicola. *Sisters in Arms: British Army Nurses tell their Story*. London: Weidenfeld & Nicolson, 2008

Veblen, Thorstein. *Theory of the Leisure Class*. New York: Penguin Classics, 1994 [1899]

Walby, Sylvia. *Patriarchy at Work*. London: Polity Press, 1986

Waugh, Evelyn. *Decline and Fall*. London: Penguin, 1975 [1928]

Webb, Beatrice. *On Keeping Well*. London: YWCA, 1918

Wharton, Edith. *The House of Mirth*. Ware: Wordsworth Editions, 2002, [1905]

Williamson, Henry. *The Patriot's Progress*. Stroud: Sutton, 2004 [1930]

Wilson, Elizabeth. *Adorned in Dreams: Fashion and Modernity*. London: Virago, 1985

Witkop, Philipp, Wedd, A. P., trans. *German Students' War Letters*. Philadelphia, PA: Pine Street Books, 2013

Woodhead, Lindy. *War Paint: Elizabeth Arden and Helena Rubenstein, their Lives, their Times, their Rivalry*. London: Virago, 2003

—— *Shopping, Seduction and Mr Selfridge*. London: Profile Books, 2008

Woodland, T. W. 'Ernst Jünger's War Diaries', *German Life and Letters*. July 1960, vol. 13, issue 4, pp. 298–302

Woodward, Rachel and Winter, Trish. *Sexing the Soldier: The Politics of Gender and the Contemporary British Army*. Oxon and New York: Routledge, 2007

Woollacott, Angela. *On Her Their Lives Depend: Munitions Workers in the Great War*. Berkeley, CA: University of California Press, 1994

Woycke, James. *Birth Control in Germany, 1871–1933*. London: Routledge, 1988

Zdatny, Steven M. *Hairstyles and Fashion: A Hairdresser's History of Paris, 1910–1920*. Oxford: Berg, 2006

Zweig, Stefan. *The World of Yesterday*. Anthea Bell trans., London: Pushkin Press, 2011 [1943]

Websites

www.firstworldwar.com
www.germanhistorydocs.ghi-dc.org
www.grandfathersgreatwar.com
www.kaisersbunker.com
www.oldmagazinearticles.com
www.ppu.org.uk
www.thegreatwar.com
www.warandgender.com

INDEX

Page references in italic denote illustrations.